Mobile Communication in Asia: Local Insights, Global Implications

Series editor

Sun Sun Lim, Head of Humanities, Arts and Social Sciences,
Singapore University of Technology and Design, Singapore

More information about this series at http://www.springer.com/series/13350

Emma Baulch · Jerry Watkins
Amina Tariq
Editors

mHealth Innovation in Asia

Grassroots Challenges and Practical
Interventions

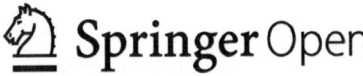 **Springer** Open

Editors
Emma Baulch
Digital Media Research Centre
Queensland University of Technology
Brisbane, QLD
Australia

Amina Tariq
School of Public Health and Social Work
Queensland University of Technology
Brisbane, QLD
Australia

Jerry Watkins
School of Communication and Design
RMIT University Vietnam
Ho Chi Minh City
Vietnam

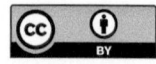

ISSN 2468-2403   ISSN 2468-2411 (electronic)
Mobile Communication in Asia: Local Insights, Global Implications
ISBN 978-94-024-1250-5   ISBN 978-94-024-1251-2 (eBook)
https://doi.org/10.1007/978-94-024-1251-2

Library of Congress Control Number: 2017958614

Printed on acid-free paper

This Springer imprint is published by Springer Nature
The registered company is Springer Science+Business Media B.V.
The registered company address is: Van Godewijckstraat 30, 3311 GX Dordrecht, The Netherlands

Contents

Contents

Editors and Contributors

About the Editors

Emma Baulch is Senior Research Fellow at the Digital Media Research Centre, Creative Industries Faculty, Queensland University of Technology, Australia.
e.baulch@qut.edu.au

Jerry Watkins is Head of the Department: Communication, School of Communication and Design, RMIT University Vietnam.
jerry.watkins@rmit.edu.vn

Amina Tariq is Lecturer at the School of Public Health and Social Work, Faculty of Health, Queensland University of Technology, Australia.
a.tariq@qut.edu.au

Contributors

Emma Baulch Creative Industries Faculty, Queensland University of Technology, Brisbane, Australia

Shreya Bhatt Medic Mobile, Mumbai, India

Huan Chen College of Journalism and Communications, University of Florida, Gainesville, USA

Arul Chib Nanyang Technological University, Singapore, Singapore

Sameera Durrani School of the Arts and Media, University of New South Wales, Sydney, Australia

Mohan J. Dutta Faculty of Arts and Social Sciences, National University of Singapore, Singapore, Singapore

Jay Evans Medic Mobile, Kathmandu, Nepal; Global Health Academy, University of Edinburgh, Edinburgh, UK

Satveer Kaur-Gill Faculty of Arts and Social Sciences, National University of Singapore, Singapore, Singapore

Chervin Lam Faculty of Arts and Social Sciences, National University of Singapore, Singapore, Singapore

Dyah Pitaloka Department of Indonesian Studies, University of Sydney, Sydney, Australia

Ranju Sharma Medic Mobile, Kathmandu, Nepal

Naomi Tan Faculty of Arts and Social Sciences, National University of Singapore, Singapore, Singapore

Amina Tariq School of Public Health and Social Work, Queensland University of Technology, Queensland, Australia

Jerry Watkins School of Communication and Design, RMIT University Vietnam, Ho Chi Minh City, Vietnam

Abbreviations

APEC	Asia-Pacific Economic Cooperation
ART	Antiretroviral Therapy
ATM	Automatic Teller Machine
BBM	BlackBerry Messenger
BHU	Basic Health Unit
CCA	Culture-Centered Approach
CDMA	Code Division Multiple Access
CDSS	Clinical Decision Support System
CE	Communicative Ecology
CHC	Community Health Center
CHW	Community Health Workers
CSR	Corporate Social Responsibility
DGM	Data Gathering Module
EMR	Electronic Medical Record
FSW	Female Sex Worker
GSM	Global System for Mobile communications
GW	General Women
HCD	Human-Centered Design
HDF	Human Development Fund
HIV	Human Immunodeficiency Virus
ICT	Information and Communication Technology
IDU	Injecting Drug User
IPA	Interpretative Phenomenology Analysis
IRH	Institute for Reproductive Health
LMIC	Low- and Middle-Income Countries
LHW	Lady Health Worker
LHV	Lady Health Visitor
MNO	Mobile Network Operators
MSM	Men who have Sex with Men
NGO	Non-Government Organization

PLWHA	People Living With HIV/AIDS
NPFP&PHC	National Program for Family Planning & Primary Health Care
RGH	Rawalpindi General Hospital
RHC	Rural Health Center
SIM	Subscriber Identity Module
SMS	Short Message Service
TBA	Trained Birth Assistant
USAID	United States Agency for International Development
WHO	World Health Organization

Chapter 1
Introduction: Social and Cultural Futures—The Everyday Use and Shifting Discourse of mHealth

Emma Baulch, Jerry Watkins and Amina Tariq

This book presents a range of studies into formal and informal mHealth initiatives from across the Asia region. The need for the book is clear—current mobile phone penetration in many Asian regions stands at well over 100% and in some cases has increased by up to 150-fold in the last 10 years (ITU, 2016). In response to this remarkable level of mobile adoption, the aim of the book is twofold: first, we wish to highlight how social and cultural research must play a more prominent role in understanding the impact of already existing, vernacular uses of mobile devices on mHealth programs. Second, in so doing, we wish to advance the research agenda for sociocultural approaches to mHealth by identifying key commonalities, challenges and points of variation manifest across the emerging body of mHealth work. The chapters in this book seek to achieve this aim by underlining the need to plan for the intricate social, institutional, political and communicative environments at the user level of a mHealth initiative. Our contributors include both established and emerging scholars as well as practitioners who have adopted sociocultural approaches within the mHealth domain. Their research highlights how an understanding of context can enable mHealth practitioners and policy makers to anticipate barriers or to perceive hitherto unnoticed possibilities that can make or break the successful use of personal mobile devices to achieve health outcomes.

Across the Asia region, mobile devices are firmly established as an essential personal item even in many low-income regions. The mobile phone is no longer considered a 'new' medium and we contend that the future of many mHealth interventions in the Asia region will no longer be about trying to changing health

E. Baulch (✉)
Creative Industries Faculty, Queensland University of Technology, Queensland, Australia
e-mail: e.baulch@qut.edu.au

J. Watkins
School of Communication and Design, RMIT University Vietnam,
Ho Chi Minh City, Vietnam

A. Tariq
School of Public Health and Social Work, Queensland University of Technology,
Queensland, Australia

© Asian Development Bank 2018
E. Baulch et al. (eds.), *mHealth Innovation in Asia*, Mobile Communication in Asia:
Local Insights, Global Implications, https://doi.org/10.1007/978-94-024-1251-2_1

behaviours via the top-down introduction of new technologies. Instead, we join a growing cadre of researchers who recommend that mHealth program designers and policy makers should seek to adapt existing user practices around mobile devices as part of their planning for new initiatives to encourage ongoing health behaviour modification (e.g. Mateo, Granado-Font, Ferré-Grau, & Montaña-Carreras, 2015). Such adaptation entails an implicit acknowledgment of the need for a diversification of research methodologies beyond conventional health research methods (Fiordelli, Diviani, & Schulz, 2013; PLoS Medicine Editors, 2013; Tomlinson, Rotheram-Borus, Swartz, & Tsai, 2013). It will also require skills in the application of social and cultural research to the design of mHealth initiatives in order to grasp and leverage the dynamic patterns of mobile usage by individuals and groups. A more detailed and site-sensitive insight into how devices, platforms and content are used at the local level will allow us to more reliably explore how mHealth innovation can achieve realistic and sustainable health outcomes. In particular, designers of mHealth interventions must pay further attention to the study of the informal processes that emerge outside—or on the fringes—of formal interventions, as mobile devices embed themselves ever further into the everyday lives of health workers, health seekers and—at times—health avoiders.

A number of scholars have investigated the potential of mobile systems to addressing structural health challenges in the region including infectious disease, mental health or lifestyle disease (e.g. Brian and Ben-Zeev, 2014; Bullen, 2013; Khatun, Heywood, Ray, Bhuiya, & Liaw, 2016). More recent academic studies address the need to attend to the intricate institutional, political and communicative environments at the local level in order to develop sustainable mHealth initiatives (e.g. Agarwal, Perry, Long, & Labrique, 2015). However, much of this work remains scattered across various domain-specific journals and books which may not embrace the cross-disciplinary approaches required by complex program design and implementation—and furthermore can be difficult to access for those outside the Academy.

Much previous work attests to a dark secret at the heart of mHealth implementation and evaluation—namely the lack of hard scholarly evidence to support mHealth's value-add to existing healthcare systems. For example, a recent systematic review of initiatives in PR China found 'little evidence of the development of mHealth initiatives that were likely to substantially strengthen health care systems' (Tian et al., 2017). This finding echoes an earlier review of mHealth initiatives in developing countries (Chib, 2013). One of the barriers to providing such evidence is revealed in the common criticism that the majority of previous published mHealth initiatives are prototypes, pilots or tests (Orwat, Graefe, & Faulwasser, 2008) which do not readily upscale to national-level systems (van Heerden, Tomlinson, & Swartz, 2012). A number of critics have attributed this limited scalability to the predominant techno-centric philosophy which underpinned early mHealth projects in the region (e.g. Whittaker, 2012; Zhao, Freeman, & Li, 2016). This philosophy can assume that technology is neutral in all contexts and therefore could be applied to specific sites and projects with limited understanding of the complexity of the underlying healthcare systems and broader cultures of communication and interaction (Curioso and Mechael, 2010). An accompanying expectation was that a successful pilot would then serve as a best-practice prototype which could be replicated across different regions and contexts with minimal adaptation, thereby achieving economies and efficiencies of scale.

While most stakeholders would acknowledge the importance of formal evidence to support client or patient outcomes from mHealth initiatives, we must also appreciate the unique difficulties in gathering such evidence. The churn of devices, tariffs, operating systems, apps, content—in short, the whole mobile consumer ecology—is so rapid that the results of multi-year studies of mobile technology interventions may be largely irrelevant prior to publication. As a result of such rapid churn, the expectation that local-level mHealth pilots can be upscaled to regional or national program level is called into question as hardware and software support for existing systems fades away, small bespoke app developers go out of business, program champions are promoted and trained mHealth staff move on to different projects. We speculate that the availability and diversity of mobile devices will push us away from the notion of scalability and towards a mHealth environment of rapid program development and implementation, in which a range of evolving user-level mHealth initiatives are deployed in a modular fashion under a regional or national health data umbrella. Within this scenario, the importance of robust, ongoing social and cultural research to underpin mHealth initiatives is clear.

Our first two chapters highlight the problems of scalability and the challenges for technology adoption by formal mHealth interventions. In Chap. 2, Tariq and Durrani report on a project funded by Pakistan's National ICT R&D fund in which lady health workers (LHWs) in rural Pakistan were trained to use mobile phones to improve field-based client data collection and interaction with remote health specialists. Using findings from in-depth longitudinal qualitative accounts from eight LHWs involved in the initiative, a range of unplanned-for barriers to implementation emerged including the extra time needed by LHWs to input data to the mobile phones over existing paper systems; and client discomfort around the storage of personal data on a mobile phone. Tariq and Durrani suggest that if mHealth 'is to be the brave new frontier in the domain of health innovations, we need to do more to understand the finer points of its contextually sensitive applications'.

In Chap. 3, Evans, Bhatt and Sharma address the issue of scalability head-on by offering a framework of nine key components to support upscaling. These include mature infrastructure, a conducive policy environment, strong institutional partnerships, well-designed and context-appropriate technology, a skilled health workforce, financial sustainability, interoperability and an evidence-based approach to mHealth. They argue that 'the key to creating a pathway to scale is to understand user needs at every level of the system and to design simple and cost-effective solutions that can have a positive impact on health outcomes' (see Sect. 2.1).

Chapters 4 and 5 examine everyday uses of mobile phones within established health outreach initiatives, in contrast to the more formal interventions discussed in the earlier chapters. They draw attention to a phenomenon that is increasingly difficult to ignore: the effect of the rapid popularisation of mobiles on those health outreach programs which continue to rely upon paper-based systems and face-to-face interaction. In Chap. 4, Pitaloka studies how a state-sponsored outreach program for diabetics in rural Java prompted the emergence of new kinds of communicative practice, specifically health-related texting among diabetic women, government health workers and volunteer assistants enabled by widening handset and network availability. Using a culture-centred approach, data collected via field-based interviews found that some of the rural women participants developed new personal communication strategies for promoting health and well-being, both of themselves and their families. Pitaloka claims that this level of behavioural change demonstrates local agency—an outcome often desired by communication for development projects.

In Chap. 5, Watkins and Baulch use a communicative ecology framework (Watkins, Tacchi, & Kiran, 2009) to investigate the use of media technologies by outreach workers in the HIV/AIDS sector in Bali and Makassar, Indonesia. Their qualitative study found that the everyday uses of mobile phones by the outreach workers were very much disconnected from face-to-face and paper-based systems for testing, treating and reporting on people living with HIV/AIDS by which the national HIV strategy of Indonesia is being executed. The authors' findings suggest that 'organic' encounters and informal mobile adoption by both health workers and clients are likely to precede formal mHealth interventions at some sites. Drawing on their interviews with the outreach workers, they demonstrate how these encounters can work to establish new layers of complexity to existing patterns of inequality in access to health services.

The final two chapters of this book take a wider and more critical view of the evolving mHealth landscape alongside the broader ideological shifts that affect discourses of health. In Chap. 6, Dutta, Kaur-Gill, Tan and Lam argue for more critical scrutiny of the part played by mobile devices in the shift for responsibility for health management from states to individuals. This can be seen in the growing use of fitness apps and devices by individual consumers, which speak to attendant processes around the commodification of health. Dutta et al. point out that mHealth scholarship is sorely missing a robust theoretical framework for examining the broader power structure in which mHealth discourse unfolds. The authors also provide a critical literature review which shows that claims for the efficacy of mobile phones in improving health outcomes are 'empirically empty' due to a striking lack of evidence. Rather, claims for the success of mHealth:

> ...have more to do with health-related finance and time-saving outcomes than health outcomes per se. For example, there are few pre-test and post-test studies to show how mHealth directly improves the health of a community. In this sense, the methodological base for claiming effects is fairly weak (see Sect. 5.1).

Chapter 7 reflects some of these issues. Whereas Dutta et al. draw attention to the creeping commercialisation of health services enabled in part by mobile phone uptake and call for a return to community consultation, Chen's chapter points to developments that complicate a mHealth landscape already featuring an increasingly powerful corporate sector. Chen studies middle-class urban Chinese fitness app users who seek out opportunities to improve their health by engaging in the privatised network of fitness app consumption and exchange. She shows how mobile devices do much more than just mediate communications between and among frontline health workers, clients and health bureaucracies in exciting new ways; they also expand opportunities for private enterprises to commodify health and to vie for prominence and validation as entities offering viable solutions to public health problems. Chen also draws attention to how the corporate commodification of health gives rise to new kinds of networks and communities, as fitness app users socialise with one another within structures afforded by app design. This chapter alerts us to the need for mHealth scholarship to pay greater heed to context not only by studying spatially bounded communities of health seekers, but also online communities revolving around health-related activities and exchanges and their inherent power relations.

In conclusion, this book recognises that mHealth initiatives cannot be executed as technical programs in a vacuum, ignoring the complex social and cultural contexts in which they are implemented. This rapid proliferation of devices, platforms and content means that mobiles are now a legacy system and any user-level mHealth initiative which seeks to modify health behaviours—e.g. by decreasing sugar intake, giving up smoking, practising safe sex—is increasingly likely to require modification of entrenched patterns of mobile phone use. The collection aims to highlight this reality. In doing so, not only do we respond to calls from mHealth researchers and practitioners for the greater inclusion of social and cultural research within the design, implementation and evaluation of mHealth programs. We also seek to stress, this research must not be limited to the documenting of 'pre-existing cultural contexts'—it should also seek to enhance understanding of how dynamic patterns of mobile usage in particular sites reshape contexts and open new possibilities and challenges for those who seek to employ mobile systems to improve health. In order to achieve this inclusion, both cross-disciplinary approaches and new conceptual frameworks derived from media and communications studies will be essential in the development of the field of mHealth research (Chib, 2013).

References

Agarwal, S., Perry, H. B., Long, L., & Labrique, A. B. (2015). Evidence on feasibility and effective use of mHealth strategies by frontline health workers in developing countries: Systematic review. *Tropical Medicine & International Health, 20,* 1003–1014.

Brian, R. M., & Ben-Zeev, D. (2014). Mobile health (mHealth) for mental health in Asia: Objectives, strategies, and limitations. *Asian Journal of Psychiatry, 10,* 96–100.

Bullen, P. A. B. (2013). Operational challenges in the Cambodian mHealth revolution. *Journal of Mobile Technology in Medicine, 2*(2), 20–23.

Chib, A. (2013). The promise and peril of mHealth in developing countries. *Mobile Media & Communication, 1*(1), 69–75.

Curioso, W. H., & Mechael, P. N. (2010). Enhancing 'M-health'with south-to-south collaborations. *Health Affairs, 29*(2), 264–367.

Fiordelli, M., Diviani, N., & Schulz, P. J. (2013). Mapping mHealth research: a decade of evolution. *Journal of Medical Internet Research, 15*(5), e95.

ITU. (2016). Key ICT indicators for developed and developing countries and the world (totals and penetration rates). International Telecommunication Union. Retrieved from http://www.itu.int/en/ITU-D/Statistics/Pages/stat/default.aspx. Accessed July 4, 2017.

Khatun, F., Heywood, A. E., Ray, P. K., Bhuiya, A., & Liaw, S. (2016). Community readiness for adopting mHealth in rural Bangladesh: A qualitative exploration. *International Journal of Medical Informatics, 93*, 49–56.

Mateo, G. F., Granado-Font, E., Ferré-Grau, C., & Montaña-Carreras, X. (2015). Mobile phone apps to promote weight loss and increase physical activity: A systematic review and meta-analysis. *Journal of Medical Internet Research, 17*(11), e253.

Orwat, C., Graefe, A., & Faulwasser, T. (2008). Towards pervasive computing in health care—A literature review. *BMC Medical Informatics and Decision Making, 8*, 26.

PLoS Medicine Editors. (2013). A reality checkpoint for mobile health: Three challenges to overcome. *PLoS Med, 10*(2), e1001395.

Tian, M., Zhang, J., Luo, R., Chen, S., Petrovic, D., Redfern, J., et al. (2017). mHealth interventions for health system strengthening in China: A systematic review. *JMIR mHealth and uHealth, 5*(3), e32.

Tomlinson, M., Rotheram-Borus, M. J., Swartz, L., & Tsai, A. C. (2013). Scaling up mHealth: Where is the evidence? *PLoS Med, 10*(2), e1001382.

van Heerden, A., Tomlinson, M., & Swartz, L. (2012). Point of care in your pocket: A research agenda for the field of m-health. *Bulletin of the World Health Organization, 90*(5), 393–394.

Watkins, J., Tacchi, J., & Kiran, M.S. (2009). The role of intermediaries in the implementation and development of asynchronous rural access. In C. Stephanidis (Ed.), *Universal Access in HCI* (Vol. 5616, pp. 451–459), Part III, Springer-Verlag.

Whittaker, R. (2012). Issues in mHealth: Findings from key informant interviews. *Journal of Medical Internet Research, 14*(5).

Zhao, J., Freeman, B., & Li, M. (2016). Can mobile phone apps influence people's health behavior change? An evidence review. *Journal of Medical Internet Research, 18*(11).

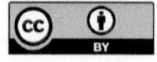

Chapter 2
One Size Does Not Fit All: The Importance of Contextually Sensitive mHealth Strategies for Frontline Female Health Workers

Amina Tariq and Sameera Durrani

Abstract mHealth solutions represent an exciting new frontier in the fight against myriad health challenges faced in the developing world, where the use of mobile phones has become pervasive across various socioeconomic boundaries. The principal users of these solutions are frontline healthcare workers; mostly women, often working at the lowest rung of health hierarchy. The distinctive value of this workforce lies in its ability to successfully deliver health services whilst being sensitive to the culture and context of their communities. Since these women are *from* the client communities, they can speak *to* them in ways outsiders cannot. Using a contextualized case study of lady health workers (LHWs) working in rural areas of Pakistan, this chapter demonstrates how the potential represented by such frontline health workers can be maximized. To this end, it draws upon in-depth longitudinal qualitative accounts of eight LHWs involved in a 2-year pilot mHealth project to improve antenatal health care. This chapter uncovers how sociocultural barriers—such as prohibitive financial concerns and gender-based discrimination—inhibit acceptance of mHealth solutions in Pakistan. The study found that these barriers adversely impact both LHWs' initial adoption of mobile devices as well their inclination to continue using mHealth solutions. This chapter explores how macro- and micro-level communication strategies can be used to ease these barriers. It also explores how LHWs themselves can use mobile technology to better connect with their client communities. If mHealth is to be the brave new frontier in the domain of health innovations, we need to do more to understand the finer points of its contextually sensitive applications. This chapter seeks to explore how this can become a reality for rural areas of Pakistan.

A. Tariq (✉)
School of Public Health and Social Work, Queensland University of Technology, Queensland, Australia
e-mail: a.tariq@qut.edu.au

S. Durrani
School of the Arts and Media, University of New South Wales, Sydney, Australia

© Asian Development Bank 2018
E. Baulch et al. (eds.), *mHealth Innovation in Asia*, Mobile Communication in Asia: Local Insights, Global Implications, https://doi.org/10.1007/978-94-024-1251-2_2

Keywords Lady health worker · mHealth · Pakistan · Context sensitive Communication strategy · Mass media

2.1 Introduction

Community health workers (CHWs) in many low- and middle-income countries are a fundamental part of the health service delivery structure (Haines et al., 2007; Maes, Closser, Vorel, & Tesfaye, 2015; Perry, Zulliger, & Rogers, 2014). A 2014 review of the role and performance of CHWs ascertains that more than five million frontline workers are active globally (Perry et al., 2014). CHWs can occupy the lowest rung of health hierarchy, work on the frontline, come from the modest social, economic, educational backgrounds, are often women, and are likely to serve their own communities (Bhatia, 2014; Haines et al., 2007; Kane et al., 2016). These frontline CHWs have been instrumental in providing a range of health services ranging from provision of antenatal and postnatal care, safe childbirth, counseling on breastfeeding, immunizations, management of uncomplicated childhood illnesses, general health education and promotion on malaria, tuberculosis, HIV/AIDs, and facilitating access to healthcare services (Kok et al., 2015; Lewis, 2010; Perry et al., 2014; Perry & Zulliger, 2012). CHWs in many cases are the first point of healthcare contact in their communities and usually have high school education (between year 8 and 10) which is supplemented with up to 3 years para-professional training (Closser, 2015; Kok et al., 2015; Lewis, 2010).

Many recent reviews of the performance of frontline healthcare workers recognize that despite limitations in the quality of available evidence, these workers have an important role in increasing coverage of essential interventions for child survival and other health priorities (Kane et al., 2016; Kok et al., 2015; Lewis, 2010; Perry et al., 2014). One distinguishing characteristic of this frontline workforce is its ability to provide healthcare services while being sensitive to the culture and context of host communities (Bhatia, 2014; Maes et al., 2015; Mbuagbaw et al., 2015; Mumtaz et al., 2013). This characteristic is part of the minimum guidelines for CHW selection set by the World Health Organization: "*CHWs should be members of the communities where they work, should be selected by the communities, should be answerable to the communities for their activities, should be supported by the health system but not necessarily a part of its organization, and have shorter training than professional workers*" (Lehmann & Sanders, 2007). As recognized by Maryse et al. in their recent systematic review, retention and performance is better in programs where selected CHWs are trusted members of the community and better reflect the linguistic and cultural diversity of the population served (Kok et al., 2015). This contextually sensitive healthcare service provided by frontline female workers is particularly beneficial for maternal care in conservative communities of the developing world (Hurt, Walker, Campbell, & Egede, 2016; Mbuagbaw et al., 2015; Mumtaz et al., 2013). Female healthcare workers—as they belong to the same community—have a comfort level with their patients, which is not possible to establish for a healthcare professional from outside the community.

Acknowledging the instrumental role of frontline healthcare workforce, various educational and technological interventions are being introduced with the intention to improve the quality of care provided by CHWs (Howitt et al., 2012, p. 508). There is growing interest in the use of mobile information and communication technologies (commonly referred to as mHealth) to revolutionize the work of CHWs in low-resource settings by providing them with efficient communication and data collection systems (Akter & Ray, 2010; Buehler, Ruggiero, & Mehta, 2013; Chib, 2013; Hurt et al., 2016; Mechael, 2009; Tomlinson et al., 2009). Partly as a result, there is a wide body of literature across many developing countries that reports on mHealth interventions with CHWs as the primary users of the mHealth technologies (Buehler et al., 2013; Chib, 2010; DeRenzi et al., 2011; Kumar et al., 2015; Ramachandran, Canny, Das, & Cutrell, 2010). Possible mHealth applications span different types of tasks performed by CHWs including data collection and reporting, information and decision support applications, and communication with healthcare professionals and patients (Chib, 2013; Hall, Fottrell, Wilkinson, & Byass, 2014).

Despite the plethora of pilot mHealth projects initiated in developing countries over the past decade, there is general agreement amongst researchers that existing evidence is rather too limited to easily permit any "scaling-up" of mHealth initiatives (Aranda-Jan, Mohutsiwa-Dibe, & Loukanova, 2014; Chib, 2013; Hall et al., 2014; Hurt et al., 2016; Källander et al., 2013; O'Donovan, Bersin, & O'Donovan, 2015; Tomlinson, Rotheram-Borus, Swartz, & Tsai, 2013). Appropriate consideration of sociocultural factors in the design of mHealth interventions is identified as one of the prerequisites to enable the much-needed shift from the pilot to a scalable mHealth paradigm. Aranda-Jan et al. suggest in their review of mobile health projects in Africa that even if pilot projects are perceived to be useful by one particular community or set of users, there are still questions regarding the acceptance of mHealth technologies by other communities, as receptiveness is limited by socioeconomic and sociocultural factors (Aranda-Jan et al., 2014, p. 12). This is further confirmed by a recent systematic review of factors effecting mHealth adoption by healthcare professionals conducted by Gagnon et al. which included mHealth adoption studies conducted both in developed and developing countries (Gagnon, Ngangue, Payne-Gagnon, & Desmartis, 2016). This review observes that along with some common factors (e.g., perceived usefulness of mHealth) across developed and developing countries, studies in developing countries identified five factors that were not mentioned in studies across developed world (Gagnon et al., 2016). These factors included professional security, support and promotion of mHealth by colleagues, additional tasks, material resources as well as communication and collaboration effort (Gagnon et al., 2016). Sociotechnical consideration of mHealth requires going beyond basic evaluation of proving mHealth works to examining the contextual conditions on what and how these solutions do or do not work (Buehler et al., 2013; van Heerden, Tomlinson, & Swartz, 2012; PLOS Medicine Editors, 2013; Tomlinson et al., 2013).

mHealth research therefore needs to shift from its techno-deterministic design focus to a contextually informed technology design focus—to ensure that technology is appropriately used in the context of achieving the specific health goals it was intended to meet (Davis, DiClemente, & Prietula, 2016; Fiordelli, Diviani, & Schulz, 2013). This shift requires diversification from both theoretical and methodological perspectives especially drawing on rich theoretical perspectives of communication and media literature (Kumar et al., 2013). Arguably, there is currently some disconnection of expertise—health professionals are qualified to say what the *content* of the messages needs to be while media professionals are better aware of the *form* these messages must take and the platforms most suitable for dissemination of these messages. We propose in this chapter that both mHealth practice and research provides important opportunities to challenge the theoretical assumptions embedded in current information systems theory, which has often been conceived within an industrial setting. The requirement now is for the development of contextually nuanced theory which is meaningful to the multidisciplinary context of the mHealth domain (Chiasson and Davidson, 2004; Chiasson et al., 2007).

This chapter brings together ideas from both domains and draws on literature that looks at the use of mobile communication as well as providing a historical overview of how mass media campaigns have been employed to support CHW programs in Pakistan. This chapter specifically aims to examine the contextually sensitive mHealth possibilities that exist within Pakistan with reference to better facilitation of communication at the interpersonal, group, and mass audience level. By drawing on a contextualized case study of mHealth implementation, it examines what type of mobile communication technologies are potentially available for frontline lady healthcare workers (LHWs) and how media can be better utilized to facilitate holistic acceptance of the LHW program as well as the technology appended to the program.

2.2 mHealth Implementation for Antenatal Care in Pakistan

This section describes a case study of a pilot mHealth project implemented in Pakistan between 2008 and 2010. Our aim is to provide appropriate background and implementation details of the project which will then be used to inform the discussion of proposed contextually sensitive communication strategies in Sect. 2.3.

2.2.1 Lady Health Workers: Primary Carers for Rural Mothers in Pakistan

In 1993, the Government of Pakistan launched the National Program for Family Planning and Primary Health Care (NPFP&PHC). This was done in order to fill the gaps created by the ever-increasing population's health needs and the deficient facility-based care mechanisms at the primary level, as well as to reduce unnecessary workload on higher level centers. The program was launched with the slogan of "*Promoting health: Reducing poverty by bridging the gap between Health Services and communities, we provide quality Integrated Health Services at the doorstep of our communities*" (Wazir, Shaikh, & Ahmed, 2013). The government program is structured around rural health centers (RHCs) and basic health units which are staffed by doctors, lady health visitors, lady health workers (LHWs), and trained birth assistants (Aqil, 2012; Siddiqui, Shah, & Memon, 2010). The program has gradually expanded since its inception and has involved more than 100,000 LHWs who provide preventive and basic curative services at the household level throughout the country (Garwood, 2006). While the term "lady" may seem rather old-fashioned to a native English language speaker, it is pertinent to note here the prestige and respect it carries within the Pakistani context of its use. It is the closest translation of the Urdu word *khatoon*, a title of respect used for an adult woman. Using the English translation as a title for these workers may have been a way of conferring further prestige and credibility onto their roles.

A LHW is eligible for employment if she has the minimal qualification of at least 5 and preferably 8 years of formal schooling. She has to be essentially a resident in the locality where she is to be assigned. This hiring is done at the district level by district health departments. The LHWs are linked with the Basic Health Units (BHU) administratively, and for referral of patients. They report to the BHU on a monthly basis and receive regular refresher training at the same venues (Garwood, 2006). Each LHW is designated to 150–200 households, or a population of about 1000. There are about 12–20 LHWs in the catchment area of each BHU (Closser & Jooma, 2013; Garwood, 2006; Mumtaz et al., 2013).

The LHWs focus on promoting healthy behaviors during the maternal period, through health education for risk of complications during pregnancy, safe practices for delivery, nutritional advice, and appropriate breastfeeding practices. A LHW is expected to: assess risk in pregnant woman based on maternal age, weight, height, and past obstetrical history; record anemia and ankle oedema and fundal height against gestational age each month; educate on the importance of tetanus toxoid vaccinations during pregnancy and on fetal movement/kicking. The LHW is also expected to refer women to higher levels of care (i.e., health facilities) if pregnancy-related complications are observed during the routine monthly household visits or are reported by the pregnant woman.

LHWs are supervised by Lady Health Visitors (LHVs) who undergo a 2-year training program that comprises 1 year of midwifery and a second year in paediatrics and tropical diseases (Ariff et al., 2010). She is qualified to conduct deliveries at household and facility level, and provides immediate newborn care. Each LHV usually supervises 20–25 LHWs. A supervisor LHV is responsible for training LHWs, and ensuring quality performance by LHWs by collecting monthly reports from the LHWs which provide information on type of cases encountered and relevant services provided (Rabbani et al., 2014, 2016).

2.2.2 Antenatal Care in Pakistan: Proposed mHealth Monitoring Solutions

To reflect on the lessons learned from the case study, the following subsections provide some necessary project background. The complete proposal of the project is available for open access from the National ICT R&D website www.ictrdf.org.pk/ (Rao, 2010).

2.2.2.1 Project Background

The project under discussion was titled "Remote Patient Monitoring System with Focus on Antenatal Care for Rural Population", an innovative 14.8 million (PKR) project funded by Pakistan's National ICT R&D fund in 2008. National ICT R&D is a government-affiliated organization which aims to *"Transform Pakistan's economy into a knowledge based economy by promoting efficient, sustainable and effective ICT initiatives through synergic development of industrial and academic resources"* (National Information Communication Technology Research & Development [ICT R&D], 2017).

At the time, the project was one of very few mHealth projects initiated in Pakistan. The primary objective of this 28-month pilot project was to develop a reliable, efficient, and easily deployable remote patient monitoring system that can play a vital role in providing basic health services to the remote village population of Pakistan at their doorstep. The aim was to design a generic remote healthcare system with a focus on antenatal care, and use ICT advancements to develop a monitoring system that could enhance the quality of health care provided by the LHWs.

In order to evaluate the performance of the project, the following performance indicators were defined: (i) LHWs' capacity, (ii) number of correct referrals, (iii) reduction in complexities in birth process through timely preventive measures, (iv) amount of correct information available during emergency cases, and (v) ultimately a reduction in infant and maternal mortality ratios in the controlled population group. The rationale of this approach was to provide a low-cost and reliable solution to the problem of provision of expert health care to patients in remote areas of Pakistan.

2.2.2.2 mHealth Solution: Overall Proposed Design

The proposed mHealth solution at the conception stage of the project incorporated the use of a remote patient monitoring system, conceived as a system which allows LHWs to fill in patient's antenatal care-related information using a mobile device. The proposed overall architecture of the system consisted of sensors for automatic measurement of patient's vital signs, a data gathering module (DGM) installed on a mobile device which allows auto-collection of vital signs data and data entry by LHWs, a clinical decision support system (CDSS) and an electronic medical record (EMR) management system accessible on any web-enabled remote terminal (e.g., a doctor's laptop). The data entered by a LHW on the device was to be transferred in real time to a doctor's computer in a hospital. The CDSS component aimed to provide timely alerts to the doctors on any data anomalies (e.g., very low Hb levels, etc.). This would allow doctors to send their feedback to the respective LHW, who would then treat the patient. Since Pakistan currently does not possess a centralized EMR solution, this system was perceived to be an enabler for long-term management of electronic data for patients, which can then facilitate longitudinal analysis of patients' health and also drive introduction of evidence-based interventions in the public health domain, which are currently and were absent in Pakistan at the time of the project. Figure 2.1 presents a pictorial view of the overall design of the proposed mHealth solution. It is important to clarify that the first pilot phase of the project, which this chapter revolves around, did not include implementation of sensors, and focused primarily on developing data gathering module for LHWs. In this phase, LHWs were responsible for manually entering the collected data into the module on their devices.

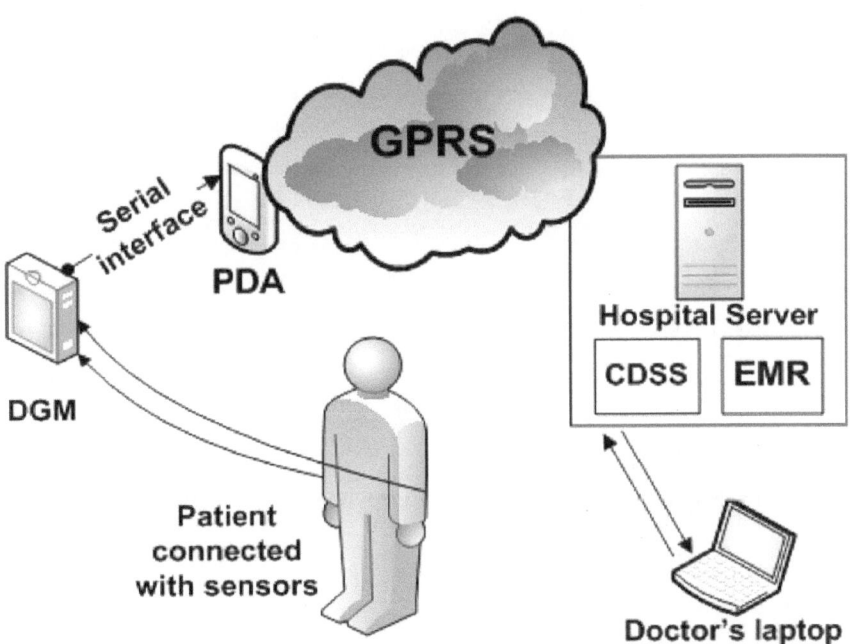

Fig. 2.1 Design of proposed mHealth solution (Khalid, Akbar, Tanwani, Tariq, & Farooq, 2008)

2.2.2.3   Project Implementation Setting

In order to better realize the practical and applied context of the project, it was essential to identify a suitable implementation setting for it. For this specific purpose, a controlled population group of pregnant women was identified, along with two expert doctors from a large teaching hospital which serves as the primary hospital to deliver care to the patients. The implementation setting therefore involved collaborative input from two key organizations: the Human Development Fund (HDF)—which coordinated the antenatal care provided by LHWs in the test region—and Rawalpindi General Hospital (RGH), a large teaching hospital responsible for providing care to the patients.

For the scope of this project, the Community Health Centre (CHC) of HDF in Islamabad rural region was targeted as it is the closest to the participating organizations in terms of geographical proximity (Fig. 2.2). This CHC is in control of one unit (comprising of 1000 households) selected from the economically disadvantaged segment of the population from rural areas of Islamabad. It was decided that the services of CHC staff (Doctor, LHV, TBA, and dispenser) would be obtained as part of the project. In order to provide expert advice on antenatal care issues, a consultant gynaecologist from RGH was also involved in the project. She

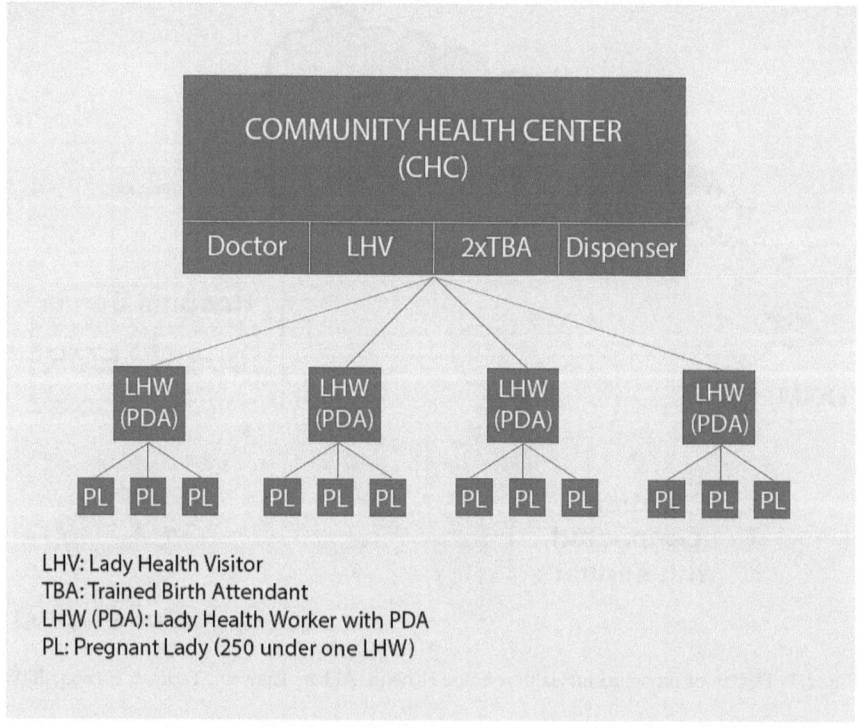

Fig. 2.2 Structure of the participating CHC site (Khalid et al., 2008)

provided assistance and expert opinion in the development of the overall mHealth solution. The hospital's approval was also obtained to enable transmission of the data to the hospital's main server, which was entered as input by the LHW using her mobile device. It was decided as part of the project plan that the electronic medical records of the patients in the study would be made available to the participating CHC as well as the National Office of HDF. The communication among RGH, CHC and National Office of HDF would be carried out through the Internet.

2.2.2.4   Project Team

The project team consisted of the following experts: a principal investigator (Professor of Computer Science), five research engineers with technical expertise in Computer Science, Electrical Engineering and Software Engineering, one medical domain expert (gynaecologist) from RGH and one usability consultant (AT—first author). The team from HDF who participated in the project included a Health Coordinator for the CHC site, a Lady Health Visitor (LHV) and all LHWs serving the CHC site (n = 8 as 6 full-time, 2 part-time). The trained birth assistant (TBA) and dispenser, as described above, were also invited to participate but had limited engagement with the project.

2.2.3   Project Implementation Journey

From the very beginning, it was clear that besides the infrastructure and associated technical challenges (e.g., quality of mobile reception in rural areas), the primary challenge of the project was to engage and train LHWs, the primary users of the mHealth solution. To address this, an initial training plan was devised around a user-centered design framework (Tariq, Tanwani, & Farooq, 2009), where a series of workshops and site visits were planned to identify LHW requirements, understand their real work context, and train them progressively as the data entry module was developed further. In order to facilitate the understanding of the project outcomes, the project journey from LHWs participation perspective can be divided into three phases: (1) requirement gathering phase, (2) initial testing and user training phase, and (3) postlaunch user feedback.

2.2.3.1   Phase 1: Requirements Gathering

The first phase comprised the first 8 months from project commencement and focused on user requirements gathering to inform system design. Requirements gathering was conducted for different parts of the project, in parallel (Fig. 2.1). This section focuses on requirement gathering for the data gathering module whose primary users were LHWs. Four user workshops were conducted: two at the participating community health center and two at the university hosting the project implementation team—to which doctors were also invited.

Contextual interviews and field observation were used to gather data to understand the context in which LHWs are situated. The age distribution of the eight LHWs was quite broad—from 17 to 58 years and their work experience ranged from 5 months to 4 years. Initial interviews revealed that seven of the eight LHWs routinely used mobile phones for interacting with their family and friends via voice calls or SMS. The LHWs' mobiles were not smartphones and did not have a camera, browser, or other more advanced functions. LHWs described very limited use of mobile phones to interact with their patients, mostly confined to informing the patient if they were late for a visit. This limited use was compounded by whether the patient had access to a mobile device and was willing to be contacted by the LHW.

A detailed task analysis identified that the main job of LHWs is to conduct periodic checkups of patients and maintain medical records. These records are documented on standard visit forms collated in a notebook primarily in English language, with occasional translation of data field headings into Urdu. The checkups are classified as "booking visit" or "routine visit". During a booking visit, the LHW logs the basic medical history of women in a new household. This history is structured as personal information, past medical history, family history, social history, previous pregnancies, gynaecological history, and general examination. During a routine visit, LHWs physically examine antenatal patients to determine the weeks of gestation, fundal height, presentation, edema, and anemia. Physiological data are measured—blood pressure, temperature, and pulse. These patient data are recorded in the paper-based register and reported back to a doctor in the nearest health center. Each LHW visits approximately 14 different households every day, meaning that a particular household is visited once a month. The average time spent by a LHW with a patient is about 5–8 min.

Each LHW carries a 5 kg bag containing notebooks and basic medical instruments. Observations and interviews revealed that LHWs were willing to adapt to a new mHealth system if they were convinced that it would improve the efficiency of their visiting schedule.

The outcome of the task analysis identified that a critical factor in selecting a device is the user-friendliness of data entry. The LHWs in this study are comparative novice mobile users and most of them used only voice and SMS features. Hence, the use of the numeric keypad for data entry was unfamiliar to them. This was further aggravated by the need to input 25–30 patient records daily. Therefore, a stylus-based touchscreen device (i-mate JAMA) was selected for the data entry module of the mHealth application (Fig. 2.3). Nine devices were purchased as part of the project, one for each participating LHW and one for project testing. At the time of project implementation the cost of each device was 12,000 PKR (approx. 110 USD).

Fig. 2.3 Custom data entry
module for the i-mate JAMA

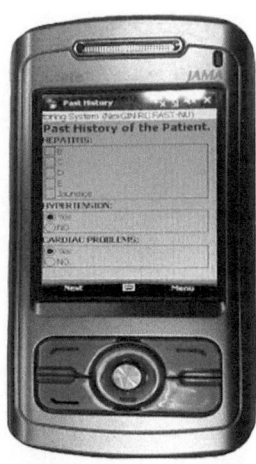

2.2.3.2   Phase 2: Initial Testing and User Training

Following requirements gathering, the project team initiated the development of the data gathering module. The design of the legacy paper-based forms (in English) was adjusted for the mobile interface (Fig. 2.3). Five user workshops were conducted every 2 weeks with the LHWs. During the first two training workshops, the LHWs mostly expressed satisfaction with the design of the form. All agreed that plenty of data entry practice would be required before field trials. The CHC coordinator and the LHV identified proposed that the LHWs enter at least 10–15 records daily for 2 months in order to gain confidence with the data entry module. This introductory training period would also allow the implementation team to iteratively test the mHealth application design.

For the third and fourth training workshops, the implementation team walked the LHWs through the data entry process a few times and helped the LHWs to enter data live while attending some patients (Fig. 2.4). The application required Internet access for data upload and the weak connection at the CHC site and throughout the rural region delayed real-time synchronization. LHWs clarified that only one of them had Internet access at home and would either need to rely on 3G service availability or visit a CHC site to upload data. The slow upload and inability to recognize if data had been successfully uploaded increased anxiety among LHWs. Based on this feedback, it was recognized that both offline storage capacity and data upload confirmation messages should be added to the system.

Three LHWs reported that mobile data entry was much slower than the paper-based entry to which they were accustomed. During the fourth training workshop, the oldest LHW refused to enter more than three fields on the data entry module as she found it very stressful and asked to be excused from the project. She

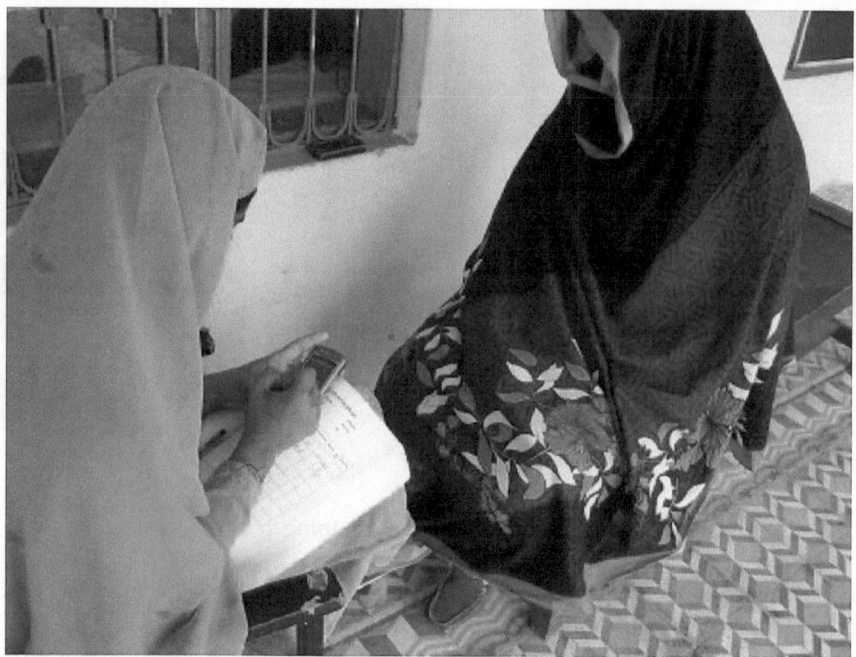

Fig. 2.4 LHW collecting patient data via mobile (Tariq et al., 2009)

was encouraged to persevere and seek help from her LHW colleagues as required. After the fourth training workshop, the devices were left with at the CHC site for LHWs to practice data entry.

At the commencement of the next workshop, it was announced that the oldest LHW was very uncomfortable with the mHealth project and had left to join a different site for work. Another LHW indicated that she intended to find another site to work at as her father did not approves of her carrying a personalized smartphone with a camera and Internet access. Four of the younger LHWs (<28 years) expressed that they really liked using the mobile application for data entry but they had been working overtime—almost four hours each day for the previous 2 weeks—to practice data entry without any financial compensation. All LHWs were concerned about being responsible for an expensive device worth almost twice their monthly salary. Those LHWs married with young children—or attending patients with young children—were worried that children's playful activities might damage the device. Others were concerned that members of their family with a substance addiction might steal and sell the device to obtain money for drugs. In response, the project investigators identified the need for an overtime budget for the LHWs; in terms of device security it was suggested that the mobiles be collected and returned from the CHC daily.

2.2.3.3 Phase 3: Postlaunch User Feedback

The final phase lasted about 7 months and centered upon full implementation including real-time data entry by LHWs, data review by hospital-based doctors, and the sharing of feedback between doctors, the LHV and LHWs. A technical support line was established for LHWs in case of any issues with the mHealth application. Most of the patient data collected via the mHealth application was received between 2:30–5:30 pm from which it was inferred that the LHWs were not using the mHealth application for data input at the patient's home as instructed, but were retrospectively entering data from paper-based records toward end of the day.

The consultant made three visits to the CHC site to gain feedback from LHWs and the LHV and to observe their use of the mHealth application. During these visits the LHV identified that she retained one of the devices (left by the LHW who left the group) for herself in case she needed to provide further training. Further feedback from the LHV indicated that some of patients and their husbands were not comfortable with LHWs using mobile devices while attending them during their visits. Therefore, most LHWs preferred taking their paper registers with them and entering the data electronically after completing their daily visits. Further discussions with LHWs revealed that—despite promises from their supervisors—they had not been financially compensated for overtime incurred on the project. One of the LHWs stated that she would leave the site soon as she found it impossible to cope with her increased workload without any extra compensation while being the sole provider for her family. The LHWs shared the reluctance of some patients' husbands to let LHWs use the devices while attending their wives as they believed it to be an inappropriate collection of private information. LHWs concerns about device theft were reiterated and there was agreement that limited effort had been made by the whole project team to create community awareness of the introduction of mobile devices to improve patient care as well as reduce concerns about data security.

2.3 The Way Forward

Both mHealth research and practice can address so-called wicked sociotechnical problem with no mechanistically deterministic resolution (Westbrook et al., 2007). mHealth projects may be characterized by abrupt stop-and-start approaches whereby a set of new measures is tested with insufficient consideration of how to normalize these interventions as part of the social fabric at the test site. This section looks at how communication practices can help to better enable sustainability with reference to mHealth. Two practices are discussed: mobile communication as a tool for enhancing the performance of LHWs, and mass communication as a facilitator for ensuring that LHWs work in a favorable environment.

2.3.1 Incorporating Communication into mHealth Programs

The case study above offers useful insights for the design a more proactive communication strategy which accounts for the evolution of communication technology in the country of implementation. The LHWs in this study did not possess smartphones—in Pakistan at this time, Nokia handsets dominated the market, smartphones were a novelty and gender was a significant factor on device accessibility within the family unit. Ownership rates have since accelerated: 53% of the adult Pakistani population now owns a cell phone, up from 5% in 2002 (Dawn News, 2015). Companies such as QMobile manufacture smartphones for the Pakistani market starting from USD 58 and estimates put the number of smartphone users at about 40 million (Baloch, 2015). There is also a generational shift: younger women—and therefore younger mothers—are more likely to have a mobile device (Qamar, 2009).

2.3.1.1 Contextually Sensitive Technological Choices

The rural/urban divide and socioeconomic disparity in this diverse customer base means that different mHealth clients in different areas will have access to different mobile devices. We argue that the concept of audience fragmentation—more usually applied to mass media forums like television (Kosterich & Napoli, 2015)—also applies to mHealth clients. In other words, mHealth project design and implementation will vary according to the demographics of the specific audience "fragment" at each different geographic site. For example, project designers may prefer LHWS to use the same mobile devices that are already prevalent at the site: if the target user has access to a phone that provides text messaging only, then it might make sense for the LHW to communicate with the same device. Additionally, the use of relatively inexpensive and commonly available devices mitigates the risk of theft, with which the LHWs in the study were very concerned.

Within the context of device use, it is important to emphasize adoption of the principle of progressive iterative familiarization in mHealth implementation. The study noted that some LHWs struggled with some aspects of the devices provided such as the touchscreen data entry keypads. An older LHW dropped out of the project altogether, while some took to using the data entry modules in a way that ran counter to project design. New technology can disrupt established social routines and so to ensure more harmonious diffusion, it is suggested that a future project take such information overloads into account. First, the technological devices being employed should be progressively rolled out so that problems encountered by users can be documented and resolved by the implementation team. Second, if the devices are similar to the type of phones that the LHWs already possess, higher adoption rates may be more achievable.

2.3.1.2   Micro-level mHealth Promotion: Benefitting from Existing Technological Options

Technology circumscribes communication, and it is therefore useful to know what kind of technology is available to client communities. The project team did not incorporate a communication plan into their project, which impacted the project's efficiency and sustainability. This section argues that communication planning undertaken with the help of professional communication advice should be made a part of mHealth project design, and proposes some ideas in this regard.

The case study looks at a rural community using non-smartphone mobile devices. This was, however, a decade ago. If a national or regional level mHealth project was to be implemented in Pakistan today, the project team would need to have data about the kind of devices that are available to specific client communities given the growing diversity in types of available mobile devices. These devices may be smartphones or older phones with limited smart features. The communication plan design will be determined by data about which technological options are available to a client community. To this end, multiple potential sources of data can be accessed by the team. Telcos and local phone retailers can provide data on devices and network usage. Social network companies may be requested to provide data on which networks are used. The team can also contact relevant officials within the health ministry, who may be able to suggest what kinds of content and media have been successfully used in which regions. This research will enable the team to design a more effective communication strategy. A communication campaign for a target LHW patch where the client community uses phones with limited features would have to rely on text messages. If they use smartphones, it may be possible to use social networking services as a messaging platform for health-related behavior change. The team could consult a local communication expert before implementing the communication plan, provided the project funding allows it.

Within a smart/mobile phone context, affordances for community-based communication contribute to two kinds of social capital, which refers to "the connections and the associated norms of reciprocity among people" (Putnam, 2001). There are two categories of social capital: bonding and bridging. Bonding social capital refers to strong-tie relationships such as family or close friends, where people share strong personal or intimate connections and provide emotional support to each other. Bridging social capital refers to weak-tie relationships such as previous co-workers or former classmates, where people do not share a similar background or emotional reciprocity (Piwek & Joinson, 2016, p. 359).

Social bonding refers to the way mobile apps can be used to build close personal bonds with family and community (e.g., Snapchat). Social bridging refers to loose networking with broader groups (a phenomenon seen within Facebook groups). Depending on the affordances of devices, health communication workers can design messages which work across the spectrum of bonding and bridging. It is possible to create group messages and updates (either text or visual message based) on a specific health issue such as advice about specific nutritional issues during a particular stage of pregnancy. These updates can be delivered to mothers, and serve as a reminder/diary. The content of these updates would be dictated by the health experts within the team and their form would be determined by the communication experts. These "diary" references can be referred to and reinforced by the LHWs during patient visits. It is a paperless and cost-effective way of delivering relevant information in a way that can be accessed by the health worker as well as the patient. While this solution will be time-intensive in design, it may assist with longer term efficiency.

It should be acknowledged that apps which facilitate social bridging will be available only to certain client communities depending on smartphone and network availability, as well as the user's level of digital literacy. This is why we suggest that a project team consults a communication expert to assist with the development of a contextually sensitive communication plan.

2.3.1.3 Incorporating Immaterial Labor Costs in Project Budgets

Although our primary focus in this chapter remains on identifying the optimal integration of communication into mHealth programs, it is vital to acknowledge that multiple actors within the mHealth system (e.g., LHWs, regional coordinators, doctors, nurses) will have to learn new skills. One prospective area of concern is the issue raised concerning unpaid overtime for the human resources involved in these projects. For instance, the LHWs included in the study noted that using data input systems cost them more time, which was unpaid. Further incorporation of mobile devices may raise similar issues, since mobile phones make it easy to work from home. A working woman, such as a LHW, is still likely to be perceived as primarily responsible for household tasks. If her work responsibilities are seen as interfering in that domain, she may face more pressure from her family in terms of performing her duties. If she is a given as a mobile device, it may contain a separate contact SIM for work only, and the LHWs can be given the option of keeping these devices on only between 9 and 5 if they wish to avoid overtime. Alternatively, the project budget should contain provisions within it to pay for overtime. We would also like to acknowledge that mHealth project owners may resist incorporating overtime costs into budgets. The research and development organizations funding these pilot projects therefore need to ensure project budgets are designed in a way that ensures that the research participants in mHealth projects are not disadvantaged financially.

2.3.2 Macro-level Strategies for Increased Acceptance of LHWs

The previous section looks at how mobile communication can help LHWs connect more effectively with their clients. This is a micro-level communication issue. However, there is a pressing need to create narratives that can help LHWs connect better with the larger society. This is a holistic, macro-level issue. The most important resource within the LHW programs are the workers themselves—technology can help improve their performance, but if their ability to work is hampered by broader social and economic frameworks, the impact of their work is diminished significantly in holistic terms. This relates again to the notion of sustainability. If the projects are to have lasting effect, the role of LHWs needs to be given more prestige within society. If the technological devices that are given to them are to have a measurable, consistent impact, their use needs to be normalized not just for the LHWs, but for their clients. The clients need to understand that the unfamiliar devices are implements intended to help them better. This kind of normalization requires the use of mass media platforms.

Human beings often make sense of their world with the help of narratives (O'Shaughnessy & Stadler, 2005). Narratives, or stories, always assign certain roles more prestige than others. The roles that are more prioritized get more attention, and are perceived as being more significant. It makes sense, therefore, for a communication or marketing campaign designer to structure narratives in a way that prioritises the roles being promoted. This is something that the LHW campaign designers did keep in mind. For culturally sensitive health issues such as birth control, it was important to first create a broader narrative of acceptance within society. As mentioned earlier, the term "Lady Health Worker" itself is an attempt to create a label or brand that evokes prestige and respectability.

The original branding efforts for the program were confined to the mass media, delivered via advertising, and television dramas. When launched in the 1990s, the LHW program relied upon extensive TV commercials, which showed LHWs visiting clients. This was an attempt to normalize a new concept: that a female worker could come to one's home, a private domain, and talk about health issues. The brand image of a stereotypical LHW was a woman in her 30s, young enough to seem modern, in traditional Pakistani garb (*shalwar kameez*, a long tunic with loose trousers) with a *dupatta* (loose shawl) covering her head. The discourse, it is noted, has been normalized enough that these ads are no longer seen as needing the same kind of airtime. Conversely, this normalization has had an unintended side effect, as LHWs have now been marginalized into the outer peripheries of media discourse and their challenges relegated to the lower tiers of media agendas.

This relegation in importance has manifested itself in economic marginalization. A string of print news reports from 2012–2016 reported on LHWs protesting about the nonpayment of salaries (as these are nonauthorial reports, see references for a list). In a 2010 episode of the talk show "News Night with Talat", prominent talk show host Talat Hussein hosted a program on the suicide of a LHW stemming from issues of nonpayment (https://www.youtube.com/watch?v=LjN3LO7D1ws uploaded 24 Nov 2010). This is an issue that highlights the importance of managing human resources, the key factor upon which this program is structured. If a LHW is impeded by finances and society from fulfilling her work, then the fundamentals on which this project rests are at risk.

This is, once again, where a communication professional may be to provide input at both the macro- and micro-level. As discussed, at the micro-level and in the short run, they can help the team to design contextually sensitive communication strategies for specific client communities. At the macro-level, they can help to support a favorable societal attitude toward mHealth and its goals. These options could relate to both traditional and social media. Access to mass audiences is restricted to some extent by considerations of finance. Access to social media, which is rapidly expanding in Pakistan, is much less restricted. For example, UNICEF Pakistan has previously uploaded LHW promotional video to YouTube to (https://www.youtube.com/watch?v=eeJTHlGM7Q0 uploaded 21 Nov 2010).

The organizations working with LHWs also need to develop better connections within Pakistani media in order to generate more news stories—like the UNICEF example above—within mainstream Pakistani channels. The change in discourse has to come from within Pakistan, from Pakistani voices. It is possible to use a two-stage process whereby blog stories written by project affiliates are picked up by influential media outlets such as *Dawn* and *Express*. One such example is the *Girls can Code* series, a collaboration between the technology forum TechJuice and *Dawn*, one of Pakistan's premier English language newspapers. A series of profile features about pioneering women working within the IT industry was penned by TechJuice writers and published on the *Dawn* website (see Rizwan, 2016a, b, c, d; Dodhy, 2016a, b). The series received positive feedback from readers and provides one template for a collaboration between a media outlet and a forum that seeks to promote female empowerment.

The case study discussed above represents an example of female empowerment within the urban context. We cite it as an example in which a human-interest angle is used to generate awareness about issues surrounding female empowerment, as well as an instance of the media partnering up with another organization to produce stories. An angle that humanizes LHWs may be one approach suitable for stories placed in the mainstream media. It should also be noted that rural health issues do make it into mainstream news. For instance, stories about infant deaths in the drought-impacted rural region of Tharparkar have dominated headlines in recent years, with coverage from regional news channels eventually making its way into mainstream Pakistani channels (Baloch, 2016). A communication strategy is required whereby awareness can be raised at regional or national levels with a contextually sensitive approach for that level, as devised by communication experts. It is also worth noting here that aside from news, TV drama series popular with Pakistani audiences represent another avenue to raise awareness about women's empowerment and their control over their reproductive rights (Haider, 2017).

The key point here, again, is that there needs to be a communication element to mHealth programs, designed and implemented by people with relevant communication expertise. As the outcomes of the project illustrate, communication needs to be improved on several fronts: between LHWs and project designers, between LHWs and their clients, and between the LHWs and society as a whole. Optimizing communication on these fronts is likely to maximize project outputs on a micro as well as a holistic level. In the long run, these practices will contribute to sustainable practices, the benefits of which will carry over successive projects. Overall our findings emphasize the need to embed communication elements within the emerging suite of sociotechnical and user-centered methodological tools (Hughes, Clegg, Bolton & Machon, 2017), which can be used as a point of reference by practitioners to help implement complex mHealth solutions.

2.4 Conclusion

This chapter brings together debates from two contiguous domains: mHealth and communication. Health care is a domain that is intrinsically dependent on communication: the ability of patients to communicate their issues, the ability of health professionals to communicate relevant solutions, and the capacity of the overarching system to effectively mediate the transmission of this information. This need to drive communication is true of mHealth as well—perhaps even more so, given that it is becoming an increasingly community-based domain. This community aspect is what makes it important to examine communication strategies from a contextual perspective. Evidence confirms that mHealth projects have difficulty continuing beyond the pilot phase and the case study discussed in this chapter has argued that contextual factors have a strong impact on project success.

mHealth projects are embedded within broader social structures, cultural and political frames that mediate how power flows within a society, hence project designs that ignore these contextual factors may be doomed. Health professionals may believe that addressing these factors is time-consuming and costly yet the eventual failure of a project is an even bigger waste of resource. This chapter seeks to initiate a debate about possible solutions to such contextual issues through the lever of communication to both identify and solve problems that imperil the sustainability of mHealth projects. It is hoped that the solutions suggested here—while far from perfect—will generate a much-needed discussion on the future design of contextually sensitive mHealth projects.

References

Akter, S., & Ray, P. (2010). mHealth-an ultimate platform to serve the unserved. *Yearb Med Inform, 2010*, 94–100.

Aranda-Jan, C. B., Mohutsiwa-Dibe, N., & Loukanova, S. (2014). Systematic review on what works, what does not work and why of implementation of mobile health (mHealth) projects in Africa. *BMC Public Health, 14*(1), 1.

Ariff, S., Soofi, S. B., Sadiq, K., Feroze, A. B., Khan, S., Jafarey, S. N., et al. (2010). Evaluation of health workforce competence in maternal and neonatal issues in public health sector of Pakistan: An assessment of their training needs. *BMC Health Services Research, 10*(1), 1.

Aqil, A. (2012). Bridging the gap between lady health workers and traditional birth attendants for reducing maternal mortality in rural Pakistan. USA: Brandeis University. Retrieved from http://works.bepress.com/anushka_aqil/1/.

Baloch, F. (2015). Telecom sector: Pakistan to have 40 million smartphones by end of 2016. *Express Tribune*. Retrieved from https://tribune.com.pk/story/953333/telecom-sector-pakistan-to-have-40-million-smartphones-by-end-of-2016/.

Baloch, S. (2016). Footprints: Death haunts Tharparkar, again. *Dawn*. Retrieved from http://www.dawn.com/news/1233906.

Bhatia, K. (2014). Community health worker programs in India: A rights-based review. *Perspectives in Public Health, 134*(5), 276–282.

Buehler, B., Ruggiero, R., & Mehta, K. (2013). Empowering community health workers with technology solutions. *IEEE Technology and Society Magazine, 32*(1), 44–52.

Chiasson, M. W., & Davidson, E. (2004). Pushing the contextual envelope: Developing and diffusing IS theory for health information systems research. *Information and Organization, 14* (3), 155–188.

Chiasson, M., Reddy, M., Kaplan, B., & Davidson, E. (2007). Expanding multi-disciplinary approaches to healthcare information technologies: What does information systems offer medical informatics? *International Journal of Medical Informatics, 76*, S89–S97.

Chib, A. (2010). The Aceh Besar midwives with mobile phones project: Design and evaluation perspectives using the information and communication technologies for healthcare development model. *Journal of Computer-Mediated Communication, 15*(3), 500–525.

Chib, A. (2013). The promise and peril of mHealth in developing countries. *Mobile Media & Communication, 1*(1), 69–75.

Closser, S. (2015). Pakistan's lady health worker labor movement and the moral economy of heroism. *Annals of Anthropological Practice, 39*(1), 16–28.

Closser, S., & Jooma, R. (2013). Why we must provide better support for Pakistan's female frontline health workers. *PLoS Med, 10*(10), e1001528.

Davis, T. L., DiClemente, R., & Prietula, M. (2016). Taking mHealth forward: Examining the core characteristics. *JMIR mHealth and uHealth, 4*(3), e97.

Dawn News. (2010a). The rise of mobile and social media use in Pakistan. *Dawn*. Retrieved from http://www.dawn.com/news/1142701.

Dawn News. (2010b). News Night with Talat-Lady Health worker commit suicide-Part-1. Retrieved from https://www.youtube.com/watch?v=LjN3LO7D1ws.

DeRenzi, B., Borriello, G., Jackson, J., Kumar, V. S., Parikh, T. S., Virk, P., & Lesh, N. (2011). Mobile phone tools for field-based health care workers in low-income countries. *Mount Sinai Journal of Medicine, 78*(3), 406–418. doi:https://doi.org/10.1002/msj.20256. Retrieved from https://www.ncbi.nlm.nih.gov/pubmed/21598267.

Dodhy, M. (2016a). Meet Noor Fatima, game developer at 'WeRPlay'. *Dawn*. Retrieved from http://www.dawn.com/news/1292593.

Dodhy, M. (2016b). Meet Sana Khan, head of digital transformation at Telenor Pakistan. *Dawn*. Retrieved from http://www.dawn.com/news/1293834.

Fiordelli, M., Diviani, N., & Schulz, P. J. (2013). Mapping mHealth research: A decade of evolution. *Journal of Medical Internet Research, 15*(5), e95.

Gagnon, M. P., Ngangue, P., Payne-Gagnon, J., & Desmartis, M. (2016). m-health adoption by healthcare professionals: A systematic review. *Journal of the American Medical Informatics Association: JAMIA, 23*(1), 212–220.

Garwood, P. (2006). Pakistan, Afghanistan look to women to improve health care. *Bulletin of the World Health Organization, 84*(11), 845–847.

Haider, S. (2017). Mawra Hocane's Sammi is a slow unravelling of one of Pakistan's darkest truths. *Dawn*. Retrieved from http://images.dawn.com/news/1177053/mawra-hocanes-sammi-is-a-slow-unravelling-of-one-of-pakistans-darkest-truths.

Haines, A., Sanders, D., Lehmann, U., Rowe, A. K., Lawn, J. E., Jan, S. ... Bhutta, Z. (2007). Achieving child survival goals: Potential contribution of community health workers. *The Lancet, 369*(9579), 2121–2131.

Hall, C. S., Fottrell, E., Wilkinson, S., & Byass, P. (2014). Assessing the impact of mHealth interventions in low-and middle-income countries–What has been shown to work? *Global Health Action, 7*.

Howitt, P., Darzi, A., Yang, G. Z., Ashrafian, H., Atun, R., Barlow, J. ... Wilson, E. (2012). Technologies for global health. *Lancet (London, England), 380*(9840), 507–535. doi:https://doi.org/10.1016/S0140-6736(12)61127-1.

Hughes, H. P., Clegg, C. W., Bolton, L. E., & Machon, L. C. (2017). Systems scenarios: A tool for facilitating the socio-technical design of work systems. *Ergonomics*, 1–17.

Hurt, K., Walker, R. J., Campbell, J. A., & Egede, L. E. (2016). mHealth interventions in low and middle-income countries: A systematic review. *Global Journal of Health Science, 8*(9), 183.

Källander, K., Tibenderana, J. K., Akpogheneta, O. J., Strachan, D. L., Hill, Z., ten Asbroek, A. H. ... Meek, S. R. (2013). Mobile health (mHealth) approaches and lessons for increased performance and retention of community health workers in low-and middle-income countries: A review. *Journal of Medical Internet Research, 15*(1), e17. doi:https://doi.org/10.2196/jmir.2130.

Kane, S., Kok, M., Ormel, H., Otiso, L., Sidat, M., Namakhoma, I. ... de Koning, K. (2016). Limits and opportunities to community health worker empowerment: A multi-country comparative study. *Social Science & Medicine, 164*, 27–34.

Khalid, M. Z., Akbar, A., Tanwani, A. K., Tariq, A., & Farooq, M. (2008). Using telemedicine as an enabler for antenatal care in Pakistan. *2nd International Conference E-Medisys: E-Medical Systems, Sfax.*

Kok, M. C., Dieleman, M., Taegtmeyer, M., Broerse, J. E., Kane, S. S., Ormel, H. ... de Koning, K. A. (2015). Which intervention design factors influence performance of community health workers in low- and middle-income countries? A systematic review. *Health Policy and Planning, 30*(9), 1207–1227. Retrieved from https://www.ncbi.nlm.nih.gov/pmc/articles/PMC4597042/.

Kosterich, A. A., & Napoli, M. (2015). Reconfiguring the audience commodity: The institutionalization of social TV analytics as market Information regime. *Television & New Media, 17*(3), 254–271.

Kumar, N., Perrier, T., Desmond, M., Israel-Ballard, K., Kumar, V., Mahapatra, S. ... Anderson, R. (2015). Projecting health: Community-led video education for maternal health. In *Proceedings of the Seventh International Conference on Information and Communication Technologies and Development* (vol. 15; pp. 17). Association for Computing Machinery. doi: https://doi.org/10.1145/2737856.2738023.

Kumar, S., Nilsen, W. J., Abernethy, A., Atienza, A., Patrick, K., Pavel, M. ... Swendeman, D. (2013). Mobile health technology evaluation: The mHealth evidence workshop. *American Journal of Preventive Medicine, 45*(2), 228–236. Retrieved from https://www.ncbi.nlm.nih.gov/pmc/articles/PMC3803146/.

Lehmann, U., & Sanders, D. (2007). Community health workers: What do we know about them. *The State of the Evidence on Programmes, Activities, Costs and Impact on Health Outcomes of using Community Health Workers* (1–42). Geneva: World Health Organization.

Lewis, J. (2010). *Busia child survival project* (Final Evaluation Report). African Medical and Research Foundation (AMREF), United States Agency for International Development (USAID).

Maes, K., Closser, S., Vorel, E., & Tesfaye, Y. (2015). Using community health workers. *Annals of Anthropological Practice, 39*(1), 42–57.

Mbuagbaw, L., Medley, N., Darzi, A. J., Richardson, M., Habiba Garga, K., & Ongolo-Zogo, P. (2015). Health system and community level interventions for improving antenatal care coverage and health outcomes. *Cochrane Database of Systematic Reviews, 12.* doi:https://doi.org/10.1002/14651858. Retrieved from http://onlinelibrary.wiley.com/. doi/https://doi.org/10.1002/14651858.CD010994.pub2/abstract.

Mechael, P. N. (2009). The case for mHealth in developing countries. *Innovations: Technology, Governance, Globalization, 4*(1), 103–118.

Mumtaz, Z., Salway, S., Nykiforuk, C., Bhatti, A., Ataullahjan, A., & Ayyalasomayajula, B. (2013). The role of social geography on lady health workers' mobility and effectiveness in Pakistan. *Social Science and Medicine, 91*, 48–57.

National Information & Communication Technologies: Research & Development. (2017). Ministry of Technology, Government of Pakistan. Retrieved from http://www.ictrdf.org.pk/beta/index.php/about-us/our-vision.

O'Donovan, J., Bersin, A., & O'Donovan, C. (2015). The effectiveness of mobile health (mHealth) technologies to train healthcare professionals in developing countries: A review of the literature. *BMJ Innovations, 1*(1), 33–36.

O'Shaughnessy, M., & Stadler, J. (2005). *Media and Society: An Introduction* (3rd ed.). Melbourne: Oxford University Press.

Perry, H., & Zulliger, R. (2012). *How effective are community health workers. An overview of current evidence with recommendations for strengthening community health worker programs to accelerate progress in achieving the health-related Millennium Development Goals.* Baltimore: Johns Hopkins Bloomberg School of Public Health.

Perry, H. B., Zulliger, R., & Rogers, M. M. (2014). Community health workers in low-, middle-, and high-income countries: An overview of their history, recent evolution, and current effectiveness. *Annual Review of Public Health, 35*, 399–421.

Piwek, L., & Joinson, A. (2016). "What do they snapchat about?" Patterns of use in time-limited instant messaging service. *Computers in Human Behavior, 54*, 358–367.

PLOS Medicine Editors. (2013). A reality checkpoint for mobile health: Three challenges to overcome. *PLoS Med, 10*(2), e1001395.

Putnam, R. D. (2001). Social capital: Measurement and consequences. *Canadian Journal of Policy Research, 2*, 41–51.

Qamar, S. (2009). Mobile phone technology growing fast in Pakistan: WB. *The Nation.* Retrieved from http://www.nation.com.pk/Business/27-May-2009/Mobile-phone-techonology-fast-growing-in-Pakistan-WB.

Rabbani, F., Mukhi, A. A. A., Perveen, S., Gul, X., Iqbal, S. P., Qazi, S. A. … Aftab, W. (2014). Improving community case management of diarrhoea and pneumonia in district Badin, Pakistan through a cluster randomised study—The NIGRAAN trial protocol. *Implementation Science, 9*(1), 1. https://doi.org/10.1186/s13012-014-0186-9.

Rabbani, F., Shipton, L., Aftab, W., Sangrasi, K., Perveen, S., & Zahidie, A. (2016). Inspiring health worker motivation with supportive supervision: A survey of lady health supervisor motivating factors in rural Pakistan. *BMC Health Services Research, 16*(1), 397.

Ramachandran, D., Canny, J., Das, P. D., & Cutrell, E. (2010). Mobile-izing health workers in rural India. In *Proceedings of the SIGCHI Conference on Human Factors in Computing Systems* (pp. 1889–1898).

Rao, S. (2010). Digital review of Asia Pacific 2007–2008. *Journalism and Mass Communication Quarterly, 87*(3/4), 659.

Rizwan, A. (2016a). Meet Bina Khan, product owner at TPS. *Dawn.* Retrieved from http://www.dawn.com/news/1296703.

Rizwan, A. (2016b). Meet Zainab Hameed, head of IT at Glaxo Smith Kline. *Dawn.* Retrieved from http://www.dawn.com/news/1296703.

Rizwan, F. (2016c). Meet Zahra Khan, team lead at software house 'Arbisoft'. *Dawn.* Retrieved from http://www.dawn.com/news/1289702.

Rizwan, F. (2016d). Meet Sara Hassan, team lead and principal software engineer at 'NetSol'. *Dawn.* Retrieved from http://www.dawn.com/news/1292593.

Siddiqui, A., Shah, F., & Memon, Z. A. (2010). Accessibility of antenatal services at primary healthcare facilities in Punjab, Pakistan. *Methods, 2011.*

Tariq, A., Tanwani, A., & Farooq, M. (2009). User centered design of e-health applications for remote patient management. In *10th Annual Conference of the NZ ACM Special Interest Group on Human–Computer Interaction, CHINZ 2009,* Auckland, NZ.

The rise of mobile and social media use in Pakistan. (2015). Avaialable at :https://www.dawn.com/news/1142701.

Tomlinson, M., Solomon, W., Singh, Y., Doherty, T., Chopra, M., Ijumba, P. … Jackson, D. (2009). The use of mobile phones as a data collection tool: A report from a household survey in South Africa. *BMC Medical Informatics and Decision Making, 9*(1), 51.

Tomlinson, M., Rotheram-Borus, M. J., Swartz, L., & Tsai, A. C. (2013). Scaling up mHealth: Where is the evidence? *PLoS Med, 10*(2), e1001382.

UNICEF Pakistan. (2010). UNICEF supports Lady Health Workers in Pakistan. Retrieved from https://www.youtube.com/watch?v=eeJTHlGM7Q0.

van Heerden, A., Tomlinson, M., & Swartz, L. (2012). Point of care in your pocket: A research agenda for the field of m-health. *Bulletin of the World Health Organization, 90*(5), 393–394.

Wazir, M. S., Shaikh, B. T., & Ahmed, A. (2013). National program for family planning and primary health care Pakistan: A SWOT analysis. *Reproductive Health, 10*(1), 1.

Westbrook, J. I., Braithwaite, J., Georgiou, A., Ampt, A., Creswick, N., Coiera, E., et al. (2007). Multimethod evaluation of information and communication technologies in health in the context of wicked problems and sociotechnical theory. *Journal of the American Medical Informatics Association, 14*(6), 746–755.

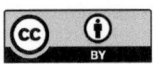

Chapter 3
The Path to Scale: Navigating Design, Policy, and Infrastructure

Jay Evans, Shreya Bhatt and Ranju Sharma

Abstract mHealth offers a unique opportunity to improve access, quality, and adherence of care in last mile and low-resource settings around the world. However, the path to scale for mHealth interventions can be complex and challenging due to the barriers presented by fragmented infrastructure, policy gaps, and more. This chapter proposes a framework of nine key components that are essential for the successful scale-up of mHealth including mature infrastructure, a conducive policy environment, strong institutional partnerships, well-designed and context-appropriate technology, a skilled health workforce, financial sustainability, interoperability, and an evidence-based approach to mHealth. While not exhaustive, this framework offers implementers and policymakers a potential path to scale up mHealth interventions in order to strengthen health systems and improve health outcomes—particularly in remote communities around the world.

Keywords Scale · Policy · Infrastructure · Human-centered design Cost-effectiveness · Data security · Integration · Interoperability

3.1 Introduction

mHealth has unearthed a unique opportunity to improve the delivery of healthcare in the most disconnected and remote regions of the world. Nowhere is this more pronounced than in low- and middle-income countries (LMICs) where health systems often face many challenges and require innovative solutions to strengthen these systems and improve health outcomes (Mills, 2014). Leveraging mobile

J. Evans (✉) · R. Sharma
Medic Mobile, Kathmandu, Nepal
e-mail: jay@medicmobile.org

J. Evans
Global Health Academy, University of Edinburgh, Edinburgh, UK

S. Bhatt
Medic Mobile, Mumbai, India

technology to address these burgeoning health systems challenges, the field of mHealth has experienced a gold rush in recent years with more than 500 distinct pilots implemented globally, many of which are in developing countries (Bjornland, Goh, Haanæs, Kainu, & Kennedy, 2012).

Despite the enthusiasm around mHealth, pathways to scale remain fraught with challenges. After the completion of hundreds of pilots, not enough is known about the uptake, efficacy, and effectiveness of mHealth interventions (Tomlinson, Rotheram-Borus, Swartz, & Tsai, 2013). Evidence shows that few mHealth pilots successfully upscale and that most often expire once the initial project funding is exhausted, with project smartphones and tablets relegated to shelves and warehouses to gather dust (Lemaire, 2011). In Uganda, for example, roughly 64% of mHealth interventions piloted in 2008 and 2009 failed to move beyond pilot stage (ibid.). There are lessons to be learned from those mHealth initiatives that have scaled sustainably which could be applied to the early stages of planning and design for scale (Hall, Fottrell, Wilkinson, & Byass, 2014). As mHealth pilots continue to grow and change the way healthcare is delivered in specific contexts, there is a pressing need for a deeper and more nuanced understanding of pathways to scale, particularly the challenges that hinder growth. For example, the Digital Development Principles Working Group provides a set of guidelines for technology-enabled programs proposed by a consortium of global organizations including United Nations agencies that can help to shape future mHealth programs (Waugaman, 2016).

In this chapter, we draw upon our own experience at Medic Mobile of deploying mHealth projects in over 23 countries in Asia and Africa, as well as available literature that supports the use of best practices for mHealth scale. Medic Mobile is a nonprofit technology company with offices in San Francisco, Nairobi, and Kathmandu that builds mobile and web tools for health workers, helping them provide better care that reaches everyone. Medic Mobile develops open-source tools that can be adapted for specific uses, backed by evidence. Medic Mobile works with implementing partners such as ministries of health and international and local nonprofit organizations, to deploy projects that leverage mHealth to improve health in last-mile settings around the world.

mHealth interventions are usually complex and their success depends upon the confluence of several factors and functions, in the absence of which scale becomes seemingly unattainable. These factors can be thought of as prerequisites and can be distilled into nine key components: Infrastructure, Policy, Institutional Partnerships, Technology, Interoperability, User-centered Design, Financial Sustainability, Human Resources, and Impact, that collectively make a "framework" for scale (see Fig. 3.1). While this is not an exhaustive list, it provides a framework to understand the challenges faced by mHealth designers and implementers in scaling mHealth interventions and hidden opportunities that may be leveraged to overcome these hurdles in an effective manner.

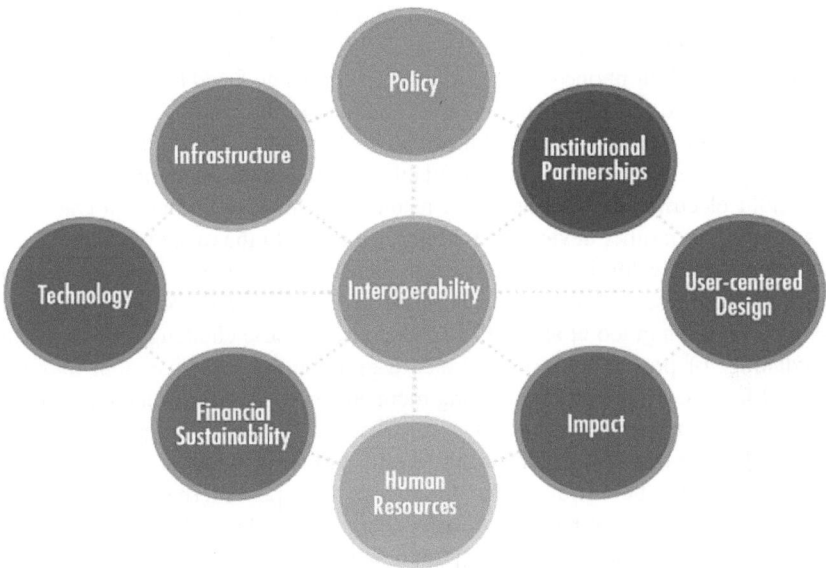

Fig. 3.1 Framework for mHealth scale

3.2   Infrastructure: Creating a Balance Between Feasibility and Sustainability

Infrastructure is one of the principal challenges to scale and sustainability of mHealth initiatives around the world, particularly in low-resource settings (Aranda-Jan, Mohutsiwa-Dibe, & Loukanova, 2014; Umali, McCool, & Whittaker, 2016). mHealth interventions are highly dependent on the available infrastructure, especially with regards to network coverage, supply of electricity, and internet access. Even though mobile network coverage is reported to cover close to 97% of the global population (International Telecommunications Union, 2015) internet access remains limited in many regions. Only 69% of the global population enjoys 3G mobile-broadband coverage and nearly 66% of the population in developing countries and 90% in least-developed countries continue to remain offline. Given the limited access in low-resource settings, mHealth interventions that do require internet connectivity for smartphones and tablets are more prone to challenges in implementation as well as limitations in their scalability (Ngabo et al., 2012).

In some countries, more people have access to a cell phone signal than to electricity (Kay, Santos, & Takane, 2011). For example, the cell network in Nepal covers roughly 97% of the population (World Bank, 2016a) but only 76% of the population has access to electricity (2016b). The population in Nepal that does have access to electricity during the dry winter season enjoys as little as 8 hours of power per day due to rationing and those hours may be distributed during nonoptimal times such as working hours or in the middle of the night (World Bank, 2011). The limited availability of electricity and its "usability"—e.g., the hours when a user can actually charge their phone—is often cited as a challenge faced by mHealth users in low-resource settings and should be considered carefully when selecting hardware during the initial design of mHealth initiatives (Chang et al., 2011). Furthermore, users may have only one or two available power outlets in their homes for all household electrical devices and as a result, they have to compete for access to these outlets with other devices and family members. In the event of limited access to electricity, mHealth users have sought other means to charge their devices such as traveling to local shops or small business, which incurs costs of travel and charging fees (Thondoo et al., 2015). In response to these challenges of access and affordability of power, users often voice a preference for devices that maximize battery life even at the cost of foregoing more advanced and multifunctional devices in favor of a simple phone (ibid.). Devices that can be easily charged within a few hours and retain that charge for longer periods will most likely have greater uptake and prove more successful in the long-term. Cheaper alternatives to charging devices such as using car batteries or solar chargers have been shown to be effective in various contexts and should be explored as potential solutions to the challenges of limited electricity in low-resource settings (Chang et al., 2011; Thondoo et al., 2015).

Our experience has shown the importance of identifying infrastructure-related challenges and referring to them during the designing and implementation of mHealth interventions. In the aftermath of the 7.8 Richter scale earthquake in Nepal in April 2015, Medic Mobile in collaboration with the Ministry of Health in Nepal deployed an mHealth intervention for daily reporting and suspected outbreak reporting of epidemic-prone diseases. The intervention was deployed in hospitals in both the urban Kathmandu valley and the heavily hit remote district of Dhading (Nesbit, 2015). The infrastructure available in these sites are very different and therefore, designing a "one-size-fits-all" mHealth tool would simply not work. While Kathmandu is a major urban center with reliable mobile phone coverage, adequate electricity for charging smartphones and easily accessible facilities for maintenance and repair of smartphones, Dhading is fairly remote with limited infrastructure. Moreover, the earthquake destroyed or severely damaged most shelters—including health facilities—in Dhading district, where 85% of the facilities were rendered non-functional according to Nepal's Child Health Division (Khanal Khanal & Lee, 2015). Road access to northern parts of the district was also cut off (Adhikari, 2015). In light of these challenges, the intervention had to be redesigned before implementation in Dhading, including the mHealth tool itself. While the community health volunteers in Kathmandu valley were able to use an Android application with internet connectivity, those in Dhading used basic phones and structured SMS, which were all that could be supported by the low-infrastructure settings of the district weakened even further by the earthquake. Health facilities in the northern areas which did not have GSM or CDMA connectivity following the earthquake submitted SMS-based reports using CDMA landline phones. Moreover, the structure of the forms on the mobile devices was also designed in such a way that it required minimal training, as health workers were trained remotely via phone calls due to the urgency of the situation and the inaccessibility of many areas. Therefore access to reliable, stable electricity and internet remain major obstacles to scale for mHealth tools that rely solely on higher end smartphone and apps requiring frequent connectivity and greater infrastructural support. Resolving these challenges requires careful design and selection of both the hardware and software to be deployed.

3.3   Technology: The Right Tools for the Right Context

The selection of hardware also shapes the future scale of mHealth interventions and can pose a challenge for the long-term sustainability of projects if not planned and executed well. Many times when launching an mHealth initiative, technological wizardry or the "bells and whistles" of new and rapidly evolving technology shape the deployment and implementation pathway rather than user needs and health priorities (Shaw, 2012). Hardware selection can also become unduly influenced by procurement and contracting guidelines created by staff unfamiliar with the limitations of settings in LMICs (Bernhardsen, 1999). Not only are newer technologies often unsupported by reliable access to network, internet, and electricity that evolve at a slower pace, but oftentimes they are not context-appropriate. Hardware used by health workers particularly in rural areas of the developing world is prone to experience excessive wear and tear over time (Iluyemi & Briggs, 2008). Ensuring the growth and long-term sustainability of mHealth initiatives then necessitates that the chosen devices can be easily replaceable or repairable in the areas where they are deployed. Corner cell phone shops or local kiosks that are ubiquitous in most small villages and towns around the world typically serve as the first point of contact for access to basic mobile hardware and repair services (Chang et al., 2011). When considering hardware for deployment in an mHealth intervention, these shops—and the devices they sell—should serve as a yardstick for the appropriate selection of project hardware. When mHealth interventions employ devices that are foreign or not easily available in local markets, they are by default harder to repair or replace in the event of damage or loss and may cause a reduction in user engagement. It is, therefore, crucial to use context-appropriate hardware that can be easily procured and repaired close to where users are located to ensure the future scale and sustainability of the intervention.

Hardware selection not only involves making decisions about the right tools for the context, but also about whether to use devices already owned by the users or provide new devices for the duration of the mHealth intervention (Ben-Zeev et. al., 2015). Benefits of using existing phones owned by users include greater user familiarity with the device and a higher likelihood that they will intuitively understand how to use the tool. However, relying on existing devices also poses several challenges. Phones owned by users may differ in their features, functionalities, carriers, and data plans. They may also be ill-suited to the specific needs of the intervention. While providing new devices to users can help to standardize the intervention across all users, it may also decrease the frequency with which the new devices are used, cause negative user experiences from having to use multiple devices for different purposes and require more user trainings, not to mention the financial implications of purchasing devices at scale for hundreds or thousands of users. New devices can also act as an incentive for users, particularly if they are allowed to keep the device after completion of the intervention, however, this may not always be feasible (ibid.).

Another factor that can influence this decision is the variance in mobile phone ownership amongst users. Not all users such as care providers and patients own a personal mobile device and often share mobile phones with family members or access the phones available to them in their community (Chang et al., 2011; Haberer, Kiwanuka, Nansera, Wilson & Bangsberg, 2010). Moreover, phone ownership rates vary significantly based on gender particularly in the developing world. There are 200 million fewer female mobile phone subscribers than male subscribers in LMICs and many women in these settings only have partial access to a mobile phone owned by male members of their family during nonbusiness hours such as evenings (GSMA, 2015). These early decisions about hardware selection based on phone ownership and suitability for context shape the mHealth intervention and can have long-lasting implications on the uptake, success, and scale of mHealth interventions.

3.4   Institutional Partnerships

Literature has extensively highlighted the importance of strong cooperation between various actors such as government, funders, and private enterprise for mHealth scale (Tomlinson et al., 2013; Qiang, Yamamichi, Hausman & Altman, 2011). These partnerships serve to incentivize and reinforce positive behaviors and are vital to create a conducive ecosystem in which mHealth can flourish. The role of mobile network operators (MNOs) in scaling mHealth interventions is particularly important (Qiang et al., 2011; Sanner, Roland & Braa, 2012). MNOs provide the architecture for implementing mHealth interventions, and as such their cooperation is crucial to the success of an mHealth deployment. However, when creating alliances with an MNO, their market share and acceptability within user populations in rural and urban areas should be taken into consideration—particularly in countries where the telecommunications industry is highly diversified (Qiang et al., 2011). The MNO landscape in India, for example, is highly competitive with more than ten MNOs offering network coverage in most parts of the country and no single MNO dominating the market. Given the competition in such settings, users frequently switch between operators in favor of those that offer the most minutes or SMS at the lowest price (Airtel, 2016). Therefore, choosing a single MNO partner for mHealth across the country in such settings becomes difficult.

A potential alternative to MNO partnerships may be to lobby for in-kind services from MNOs by leveraging government or physician membership organization relationships. An example of this is Switchboard, a nonprofit organization that has successfully created a free calling network for healthcare providers in Ghana and Liberia (Switchboard, 2017). The network not only benefits health systems in these countries by facilitating free communication and coordination between care providers in rural and urban health centers, but also serves to build MNO brand loyalty among users and increases the participating MNOs' consumer base as healthcare providers increasingly use the same operators for their personal use. Incentivizing MNOs to dedicate free or reduced cost SMS, data, and call facilities may be a more effective long-term strategy for mHealth scale and sustainability rather than relying on partnership agreements with a single operator. Innovative partnerships that create incentives and positively change stakeholder behaviors, therefore, are crucial for the success and scale of mHealth interventions.

3.5   Human Resources

The crucial components of infrastructure for mHealth scale and sustainability are not just limited to the availability of context-appropriate hardware, a cell phone tower, and an active power source but also include human resource infrastructure in the form of a skilled health workforce. In many LMICs, the cadre of community health workers (CHWs) may have achieved only basic literacy levels via formal schooling and typically have no tertiary education (Lehmann & Sanders, 2007). Health professionals need to be educated on the potential role of technology in healthcare delivery in order to achieve and sustain mass adoption of mHealth (Mechael et al., 2010). While CHWs in LMICs receive standard training on topics such as general health and basic record-keeping, such training should not be assumed to include indoctrination into mHealth (Lehmann & Sanders, 2007). CHWs and other healthcare personnel may already own and be familiar with using cell phones but they may not be well-versed with specific features and are often not fully prepared or equipped to use those same devices for an mHealth project (Ben-Zeev et al., 2015). In order for CHWs to start thinking of and using their mobiles as communication and coordination tools for health activities that form part of a ministry of health information system, they must have adequate and context-relevant training in technology (Mechael et al., 2010). Given the variance in skill sets and levels of literacy among CHWs, there is a need for continuous support and training to maintain their effective contribution not only in their healthcare knowledge but also in technology and its use (Lehmann & Sanders, 2007). Refresher mHealth training for CHWs have been effective in addressing observed technology usability gaps and improving impact during an intervention and can also contribute significantly to long-term project sustainability and scale (Modi et al., 2015; Haberer et al., 2010). mHealth training is not only essential for users such as healthcare providers but also for other key actors in an mHealth ecosystem such as project managers, application developers, and information technology specialists who require training in the development and maintenance of platforms including software and hardware to support mHealth implementations locally (Chetley, Davies, Trude, McConnell & Ramirez, 2006; Aranda-Jan et al., 2014). Therefore, a health workforce skilled in the use and maintenance of technology is a prerequisite for the success and scale of technology interventions.

A related barrier to the scale of mHealth interventions is continued engagement and motivation of health workers over the duration of the project and in the longer run. While users may be motivated at the start of a project, experience suggests that this motivation may often wane over longer periods of time (Haberer et al., 2010). Although research on CHW motivation as a result of mHealth is limited, there is some evidence to suggest that being more efficient and effective in their work tasks by virtue of mHealth is motivating for CHWs (Strachan et al., 2012). To the extent that mHealth interventions can continue to enhance health worker efficiency, CHWs will remain motivated to engage with the technology platforms for longer periods of time. Beyond efficiency, CHWs also respond to a sense of being valued by the communities they serve and the health systems they work within. A motivational technique that the mHealth system in Nepal uses, for instance, is a simple "thank you" text message delivered to CHWs after they perform certain activities such as registering a new pregnancy on their mobile device; this has been found to improve and sustain CHW motivation levels over time (Sharma et al., 2015).

Experience also shows that mHealth training for CHWs and the resulting improvement in their skill set leads to greater health worker confidence, motivation, and enthusiasm to participate in mHealth interventions (Haberer et al., 2010). Continuous training during mHealth deployments, therefore, is important to not only update knowledge and skills but also to maintain health worker enthusiasm levels throughout the duration of the project and beyond. Finally, several mHealth initiatives have also found that providing minor financial incentives such as airtime credit motivates CHWs and ensures their continued participation and uptake of technology (ibid.; Lester et al., 2010). When planning and designing for scale, mHealth interventions that can budget for such incentives for health workers over the life of the deployment stand a greater chance of long-term CHW engagement and therefore success.

3.6 Policy

The national policy and regulatory landscape—particularly an LMIC—is essential for mHealth scale and sustainability. The lack of guiding policies from the government is frequently cited as a major reason for the failure of mHealth programs (Leon, Schneider & Daviaud, 2012; Aranda-Jan et al., 2014). When an LMIC government defines an mHealth and wider eHealth strategy—including clearly established standards for data security and interoperability—and is willing to facilitate the integration of mHealth initiatives into the existing healthcare system, the mHealth systems in that country are more likely to be sustained (Aranda-Jan et al., 2014; Lemaire, 2011). While a significant proportion of countries have recognized this and more than half of WHO member states have already adopted a broader eHealth strategy within which national mHealth programs can be ensconced (World Health Organization, 2016) much more remains to be done. In a recent WHO survey, the lack of legal regulation was cited as one of the top two barriers to mHealth (ibid.). Much of the need for legal regulation around mHealth in LMICs stems from data privacy and confidentiality concerns.

Traditional paper-based systems of healthcare inherently pose a data privacy risk which can be mitigated by electronic health records and care coordination systems such as mHealth. As a result, mHealth and the broader eHealth ecosystem are often framed as "safe" mechanisms to facilitate and provide health service delivery. However, governments must define and impose comprehensive legal provisions to ensure that the storage and exchange of information over electronic methods are truly safe, particularly, in LMICs where mHealth platforms are already beginning to flourish. Legislation alone, however, is not the solution. Experience has shown that even when mHealth legislation exists, public misinformation may, in fact, derail an mHealth project (Eysenbach, 2009). Therefore, governments not only need to create and implement appropriate legislation, but also put in place a regulatory authority or body to monitor mHealth initiatives within a country. In the absence of both clearly established legislation and a regulatory authority, the integrity and credibility of any new mHealth tool may be jeopardized.

While government institutions have programmatic authority to evaluate mHealth initiatives, the lack of legislative authority with the knowledge to execute fair judgment may render their mHealth evaluations baseless and ineffective, hindering the scale of such programs. Moreover, the interpretation of the newly passed regulations may face challenges in courts where judges presiding over such cases may not have sufficient experience adjudicating cases related to technology (Timm, 2014). In such cases, a regulatory authority overseeing mHealth programs may be able to lend their expertise and knowledge to bring such cases to a just culmination. It is equally important to note that while some states have passed complete sets of regulations that are intended to govern mHealth within their borders, there are many times poor coordination among competing government ministries and agencies in charge of the oversight and management of the mHealth space (Lemaire, 2011). The same can be true among different departments managing various verticals within a ministry of health. Given such challenges, the mHealth authority in the country must also take on the coordination around policy and legislation among relevant ministries and sectors (ibid.).

The mHealth landscape in a country is not only affected by its own policy and regulatory environment, but also by the policy and regulatory settings of its neighbors the surrounding region. Policies and legislation on mHealth in LMICs, as well as developed countries, tend to vary a great deal. For example, regulations on spam advertising to mobile phones and privacy policies for smartphone apps—as well as what these policies are allowed to include—often vary significantly from country to country even within the same region such as South Asia or East or West

Africa. Significant variations exist in policies and regulations around mHealth even in countries belonging to the same geographical region, which may negatively affect mHealth scale across borders (World Health Organization, 2016). Moreover, few standards exist for data confidentiality and sharing among countries within geographical regions, which further hinders mHealth scale across borders (ibid.).

In an ideal scenario, all relevant mHealth-related policies are well-established and institutionalized by the time an mHealth initiative is ready to scale. However, the current reality is that many LMICs are still in the process of developing or refining such policies, and the speed of maturity of mHealth initiatives and supporting public policies do not match. Even if the framework legislation has been established, the regulatory environment that must accompany laws on mHealth is simply not present in many LMICs. Given this, mHealth systems must also, for the time being, address such gaps. Aligning an mHealth tool to fit within the confines of a nascent regulatory structure means that the tool must also be flexible enough to change and adapt to new regulations as they emerge. At times this may mean establishing the capacity for ongoing design evaluation during or after a successful small-scale pilot of the tool. Deploying within a country where the regulatory framework around mHealth may not be fully developed will also demand more time dedicated to building and maintaining relationships with the Ministry of Health and other ministries involved in the governance of digital health. Failure to actively engage government ministries may result in projects being delayed, abandoned, or outright banned (Eckman, Gorski & Mehta, 2016).

mHealth scale cannot be achieved in the absence of an effective policy and regulatory environment and there are some immediate steps that can be taken to achieve this. LMIC governments must adopt appropriate legislation and establish a regulatory authority to create a framework within which mHealth initiatives can flourish. Simultaneously—at the global community level—international efforts must focus on identifying best policy practices that enable and promote mHealth adoption and innovation particularly in low-resource settings (World Health Organization, 2016).

3.7   Financial Sustainability

3.7.1   Direct Government Financing

Lack of funding is one of the top reasons for the premature discontinuation of potentially valuable mHealth initiatives (World Health Organization, 2016). Moreover, empirical evidence also suggests that health technology projects often cost more than initially planned, imposing additional financial pressures during the life of a project (Leon et al., 2012). In most countries, government funding commitment to an mHealth initiative is critical to ensuring its continuity as an integrated component within an existing health system. As discussed above, well-established mHealth governance mechanisms, comprehensive evidence to supporting the mHealth system and ground level consensus on the value and credibility of the system are all critical in guaranteeing government funding. Furthermore, the timelines for national planning and budgeting need to be considered and planned for accordingly. The government needs to be prepared to propose new inclusions into national budgets well before the new fiscal year is set to begin or any periodic plans are being formulated. Even though a national health budget might be governed by a health ministry, the budget requires approval from a finance ministry. Hence communication between the health and finance ministries is critical to the budget approval process and this requires the health ministry to speak the same language as their colleagues in finance; just being enthusiastic about a new mHealth initiative will not be sufficient.

3.7.2   Alternative Ways of Sustainable Financing

Financing does not only imply assigning budgets for required line items. There are various ways that a government might finance any mHealth initiative— getting subsidies for SMS, data, and voice calls is one of the most relevant ways. Government is usually the most appropriate agency to request MNOs in a given country to provide subsidies for mHealth initiatives; such a request is easiest for MNOs to process when it involves specific professional groups of health workers. An example of this is the partnership between the Rwandan Ministry of Health and MNOs that resulted in a ten-fold reduction in the cost per SMS for a mHealth pilot to improve maternal and child health in the country, which was crucial in planning for the project's expansion and ensuring its long-term sustainability (Ngabo et al., 2012).

Building components of mHealth foundational and continuing training into an existing national curriculum for health workers can be an efficient way to finance a major component of most mHealth initiatives. Operational costs such as personnel salaries and initiatives, hardware and software maintenance or update can also be absorbed into regular program budgets. In addition, buy-in and ownership of the community that is most intimately impacted by the mHealth initiative may attract some portion of direct funding as well as provide evidence of system uptake.

3.7.3   Cost-Effectiveness

A major barrier to scale for mHealth interventions is their perceived cost-effectiveness versus paper-based systems that they are intended to replace. Insufficient evidence exists about the cost-effectiveness of mHealth interventions as many evaluations focus on feasibility and user acceptance rather than cost. Where information on costs is available, it can be limited and difficult to interpret due to subsidies in technology (Zurovac et al., 2011; Leon et al., 2012). Designing for scale and sustainability requires an understanding of the various elements that make up the total cost of an mHealth intervention including developing and maintaining platforms, training and retraining users, procuring and replacing hardware as well as ongoing data and SMS costs. Opportunities exist in each of these elements to improve the overall cost-effectiveness of an mHealth intervention, particularly at scale.

When it comes to developing systems, leveraging open-source platforms that are freely available and reusable rather than proprietary systems help to lower costs significantly, especially for future redesign, implementation, and scale (Rajput et al., 2012). Hardware costs can be a particularly daunting challenge. While the costs of smartphones in both developed and LMIC markets are rapidly declining making advanced mobile devices more widely available to greater proportion of the population (The Economist, 2014), procuring handsets at scale can pose a significant initial investment and requires financial support and subsidies to enhance cost-effectiveness of the intervention (Qiang et al., 2011). Moreover, mobile devices are often prone to theft, loss or damage in LMIC settings and costs to repair or replace devices at scale can be prohibitive (Chang et al., 2011). Strategies to curb costs of purchasing new devices may include using locally available entry-level phones (Leon et al., 2012), designing flexible, device-agnostic systems that can work on a range of mobile devices and facilitate the selection of least expensive hardware for future implementation (Rajput et al., 2012) or leveraging personal phones of users, keeping in mind the potential shortcomings of such a choice. The ongoing costs of mHealth intervention include data, voice, and SMS charges and while these rates can be quite low in many LMICs, significant budgeting and funding is required to meet these ongoing cost components at project scale where thousands of users are required to send text messages or make calls on a daily basis. Hence the importance of strategies which lower these ongoing costs such as private–public partnerships between government and private MNOs as mentioned earlier.

A frequent question concerns the cost-effectiveness of replacing existing paper-based systems with expensive mHealth systems. Earlier research indicates that standard paper-based systems can incur hidden costs in terms of staff time to maintain and correct data entry errors and/or the storage of paper records that are often overlooked when assessing cost-effectiveness (Tomlinson et al., 2009; Holeman & Nesbit, 2010). Addressing this cost barrier to implementation and scale calls for further evidence-based research into the cost-effectiveness of mHealth interventions compared to traditional paper-based systems and/or hybrid systems which combine electronic and paper-based systems. Establishing the cost-effectiveness of mHealth implementation is indispensable to support the argument for the scale and long-term sustainability of mHealth.

3.8 Interoperability: An Open Architecture Framework

Interoperability is a buzzword that is frequently exchanged at most global forums on mHealth, and much has been documented about the importance of building platforms that can communicate and integrate with existing systems of care as a way to ensure future scale and sustainability (van Heerden, Tomlinson & Swartz, 2012; PLOS Medicine Editors, 2013). Traditionally health information systems have been built using a silo approach wherein devices and disease-specific applications cannot easily share data with one another. However, there is a growing recognition of the need for improved data integration (De Maeseneer, van Weel, Egilman, Demarzo & Sewankambo, 2012) alongside interoperable health technology (van Heerden et al., 2012). National-level systems such as the open-source District Health Information Software 2 are currently used in multiple countries for routine health data collection, reporting, and management (DHIS2, n.d.). It is likely that this kind of open source and interoperable mHealth system can have a much greater chance of long-term sustainability rather than parallel siloed solutions. In terms of architecture interoperability, OpenHIE has developed a three-layer health information architecture framework which connects external systems and actors to multiple health datasets via an interoperability services layer (OpenHIE, n.d.). When successfully implemented, these kinds of open architectures can act as an "innovation infrastructure" in the same way as a mobile network or an electricity grid, enhancing the potential power and impact of mHealth systems (Estrin & Sim, 2010). Government, industry, and donors need to, therefore, cooperate and adopt an open architecture-based approach to developing and implementing mHealth interventions in order to ensure their success, scale, and long-term sustainability.

3.9 User-Centered Design

Allotting time and resources to product and project design for mHealth initiatives can yield positive results as the solution scales from a pilot project up to state, district, or national level (Eckman et al., 2016). Technology is the only component of this design challenge; attention must also be given to the end users of the system—usually a health worker—and how a new tool will help them. Those mHealth projects that incorporate user-centered design principles from the outset can fare better than those that did not (Eckman et al., 2016).

Medic Mobile has employed Human-Centered Design (HCD), a specific user-centered design approach that emphasizes a deep understanding of human capabilities, motivations, concerns, and values as they consistently surface in their daily lives; the reliability of a new technology is determined by the routine actions of users within the system (Bannon, 2011). HCD is more a way of thinking than a defined procedure and can take various shapes based on the context and the methods used to put this approach into practice (Kane, 2016).

3.10   Impact

While the global health community—including NGOs, governments, and donors—continues to display some enthusiasm for mHealth, the lack of rigorous program evaluations presents a barrier to quality mHealth implementations (PLOS Medicine Editors, 2013; Tamrat & Kachnowski, 2012). The multiyear timeframe required for this kind of program evaluation means that the technology and systems under investigation may have become obsolete by the time that findings are published (Kumar et al., 2013). Therefore, the field of mHealth may benefit from other forms of supporting evidence via continuous monitoring of program activity and outcomes to inform timely dissemination of lessons learned and best practices. The inclusion of robust monitoring and evaluation components within program design is of utmost importance to scaling mHealth systems (ibid.; Agarwal et al., 2016; Whittaker, Merry, Dorey & Maddison, 2012).

3.11   Conclusion: The Path to Scale

mHealth offers an unprecedented opportunity to reach last mile populations around the world and improve health outcomes in challenging settings. However, mHealth interventions are often complex and messy and the narrative around their scale can attract skepticism. Nevertheless, a number of successful mHealth tools and projects have followed a viable pathway from pilot to scale and lessons from these can guide governments, funders, and private enterprise to shape the future mHealth landscape. Albeit challenging, mHealth scale can be achieved with a favorable overarching framework of infrastructure, regulatory and policy environment, stakeholder partnerships, and financial sustainability; as well as a focus on interoperability, context-appropriate technology, robust user-centered design, a skilled health workforce, and an impact-driven approach to mHealth. This checklist offers a potential path to scale that can enable mHealth to fulfill its promise of strengthening systems and improving health outcomes, particularly in low-resource settings.

References

Adhikari, K. (2015, July 13). Lack of road connection keeps quake-hit Dhading folks in trouble. *The Himalayan Times*. Retrieved from https://thehimalayantimes.com/nepal/lack-of-road-connection-keeps-quake-hit-dhading-folks-in-trouble. Accessed 28 Feb 2017.

Agarwal, S., LeFevre, A. E., Lee, J., L'Engle, K., Mehl, G., Sinha, C., et al. (2016). Guidelines for reporting of health interventions using mobile phones: Mobile health (mHealth) evidence reporting and assessment (mERA) checklist. *BMJ, 352,* i1174.

Airtel. (2016). *Customer Churn*. Retrieved from iCreate website. http://www.airtel.in/icreate/common/files/iCreate_Finance_case_study_2016.pdf. Accessed 5 Jan 2017.

Aranda-Jan, C. B., Mohutsiwa-Dibe, N., & Loukanova, S. (2014). Systematic review on what works, what does not work and why of implementation of mobile health (mHealth) projects in Africa. *BMC Public Health, 14*(1), 188.

Bannon, L. (2011). Reimagining HCI: Toward a more human-centered perspective. *Interactions, 18*(4), 50–57.

Ben-Zeev, D., Schueller, S. M., Begale, M., Duffecy, J., Kane, J. M., & Mohr, D. C. (2015). Strategies for mHealth research: Lessons from 3 mobile intervention studies. *Administration and Policy in Mental Health and Mental Health Services Research, 42*(2), 157–167.

Bernhardsen, T. (1999). Choosing a GIS. *Geographical. Information Systems, 2,* 589–600.

Bjornland, D., Goh, E., Haanæs, K., Kainu, T., & Kennedy, S. (2012). *The Socio-economic impact of mobile health.* The Boston Consulting Group.

Chang, L. W., Kagaayi, J., Arem, H., Nakigozi, G., Ssempijja, V., Serwadda, D., ...Reynolds, S. J. (2011). Impact of a mHealth intervention for peer health workers on AIDS care in rural Uganda: A mixed methods evaluation of a cluster-randomized trial. *AIDS and Behavior, 15*(8) (1776).

Chetley, A., (Ed.). Davies, J., Trude, B., McConnell, H., Ramirez, R., Shields, T., ... Nyamai-Kisia, C. (2006). *Improving health, connecting people: The role of ICTs in the health sector of developing countries—A framework paper.* InfoDev Working Paper, no. 7. Health. Washington, DC: World Bank. Retrieved from http://documents.worldbank.org/curated/en/234041468163474585/Improving-health-connecting-people-the-role-of-ICTs-in-the-health-sector-of-developing-countries-a-framework-paper.

De Maeseneer, J., van Weel, C., Egilman, D., Demarzo, M., & Sewankambo, N. (2012). Tackling NCDs: A different approach is needed–authors' reply. *The Lancet, 379*(9829), 1873–1874.

DHIS2 (n.d.). *DHIS2*. Retrieved from (DHIS2) District Health Information Software website. http://dhis2.org. Accessed 4 Jan 2017.

Eckman, M., Gorski, I., & Mehta, K. (2016). Leveraging design thinking to build sustainable mobile health systems. *Journal of Medical Engineering & Technology, 40*(7–8), 422–430.

Estrin, D., & Sim, I. (2010). Open mHealth architecture: An engine for health care innovation. *Science, 330*(6005), 759–760.

Eysenbach, G. (2009). Infodemiology and infoveillance: Framework for an emerging set of public health informatics methods to analyze search, communication and publication behavior on the internet. *Journal of Medical Internet Research, 11*(1), e11.

GSMA. (2015). *Bridging the gender gap: Mobile access and usage in low and middle-income countries.* Retrieved from Group Speciale Mobile Association (GSMA) website. http://www.gsma.com/mobilefordevelopment/wp-content/uploads/2016/02/Connected-Women-Gender-Gap.pdf. Accessed 3 Jan 2017.

Haberer, J. E., Kiwanuka, J., Nansera, D., Wilson, I. B., & Bangsberg, D. R. (2010). Challenges in using mobile phones for collection of antiretroviral therapy adherence data in a resource-limited setting. *AIDS and Behavior, 14*(6), 1294–1301.

Hall, C. S., Fottrell, E., Wilkinson, S., & Byass, P. (2014). Assessing the impact of mHealth interventions in low-and middle-income countries–What has been shown to work? *Global Health Action, 7.*

Holeman, I., & Nesbit, J. (2010). mHealth basics and human scalability. *Harvard College Global Health Review, 11*(1), 40–43.

Iluyemi, A., & Briggs, J. S. (2008). *Technology matters!: Sustaining eHealth in developing countries: Analyses of mHealth innovations.* Institution of Engineering and Technology (IET).

International Telecommunications Union (2015, May). *ICT facts & figures: The world in 2015,* pp. 1–6. Retrieved from https://www.itu.int/en/ITU-D/Statistics/Documents/facts/ICTFactsFigures2015.pdf. Accessed 5 Jan 2017.

Kane, D. (2016, March 31). Medic mobile's human-centered design toolkit: A spotlight on sketch cards [Blog post]. *Medic Mobile Blog.* Retrieved from http://medicmobile.org/blog/medic-mobiles-human-centered-design-toolkit-a-spotlight-on-sketch-cards. Accessed 8 Jan 2017.

Kay, M., Santos, J., & Takane, M. (2011). mHealth: New horizons for health through mobile technologies. *World Health Organization, 3,* 66–71.

Khanal, V., Khanal, P., & Lee, A. H. (2015). Sustaining progress in maternal and child health in Nepal. *The Lancet, 385*(9987), 2573.

Kumar, S., Nilsen, W.J., Abernethy, A., Atienza, A., Patrick, K., Pavel, M., …Hedeker, D. (2013). Mobile health technology evaluation: The mHealth evidence workshop. *American Journal of Preventive Medicine, 45*(2), 228–236.

Lehmann, U., & Sanders, D. (2007). *Community health workers: What do we know about them. The state of the evidence on programmes, activities, costs and impact on health outcomes of using community health workers* (pp. 1–42). Geneva: World Health Organization.

Lemaire, J. (2011). *Scaling up mobile health: Elements necessary for the successful scale up of mHealth in developing countries.* Geneva: Advanced Development for Africa.

Leon, N., Schneider, H., & Daviaud, E. (2012). Applying a framework for assessing the health system challenges to scaling up mHealth in South Africa. *BMC Medical Informatics and Decision Making, 12*(1), 123.

Lester, R.T., Ritvo, P., Mills, E.J., Kariri, A., Karanja, S., Chung, M.H., …Marra, C.A. (2010). Effects of a mobile phone short message service on antiretroviral treatment adherence in Kenya (WelTel Kenya 1): A randomised trial. *The Lancet, 376*(9755), 1838–1845.

Mechael, P., Batavia, H., Kaonga, N., Searle, S., Kwan, A., Goldberger, A., …Ossman, J. (2010). *Barriers and gaps affecting mHealth in low and middle-income countries: Policy white paper* (pp. 1–79). Columbia University. Earth Institute. Center for Global Health and Economic Development (CGHED): With mHealth Alliance.

Mills, A. (2014). Health care systems in low- and middle-income countries. *New England Journal of Medicine, 370*(6), 552–557.

Modi, D., Gopalan, R., Shah, S., Venkatraman, S., Desai, G., Desai, S., & Shah, P. (2015). Development and formative evaluation of an innovative mHealth intervention for improving coverage of community-based maternal, newborn and child health services in rural areas of India. *Global Health Action, 8.*

Nesbit, J. (2015, June 23). Response and rebuilding health systems in Nepal [Blog post]. *Medic Mobile Blog.* Retrieved from http://medicmobile.org/blog/nepal-earthquake-how-you-can-help. Accessed 28 Feb 2017.

Ngabo, F., Nguimfack, J., Nwaigwe, F., Mugeni, C., Muhoza, D., Wilson, D.R., …Binagwaho, A. (2012). Designing and implementing an innovative SMS-based alert system (RapidSMS-MCH) to monitor pregnancy and reduce maternal and child deaths in Rwanda. *Pan African Medical Journal, 13*(31).

OpenHIE (n.d.). *Architecture.* Retrieved from Open Health Information Exchange (OHIE) website ohie.org/architecture/. Accessed 4 Jan2017.

PLOS Medicine Editors (2013). A reality checkpoint for mobile health: Three challenges to overcome. *PLoS Med, 10*(2), e1001395.

Qiang, C. Z., Yamamichi, M., Hausman, V., & Altman, D. (2011). *Mobile applications for the health sector.* Washington: World Bank.

Rajput, Z. A., Mbugua, S., Amadi, D., Chepnġeno, V., Saleem, J. J., Anokwa, Y., …Were, M.C. (2012). Evaluation of an android-based mHealth system for population surveillance in developing countries. *Journal of the American Medical Informatics Association, 19*(4), 655–659.

Sanner, T. A., Roland, L. K., & Braa, K. (2012). From pilot to scale: Towards an mHealth typology for low-resource contexts. *Health Policy and Technology, 1*(3), 155–164.

Sharma, R., Harsha, A., Acharya, P., Okada, E., Yangdol, T., Bhatta, S., ...Dahal, S. (2015). Pilot and evaluation of the feasibility SafeSIM: A mobile technology platform for maternal health care coordination in Nepal. *Publication Timeline*: TBD.

Shaw, V. (2012). Measuring the impact of e-health. *Bulletin of the World Health Organization, 90,* 326–327.

Strachan, D. L., Källander, K., ten Asbroek, A. H., Kirkwood, B., Meek, S. R., Benton, L., ...Hill, Z. (2012). Interventions to improve motivation and retention of community health workers delivering integrated community case management (iCCM): Stakeholder perceptions and priorities. *The American Journal of Tropical Medicine and Hygiene, 87*(5), 111–119.

Switchboard. (2017). Work. Retrieved from switchboard.org/work. Accessed 4 Jan 2017.

Tamrat, T., & Kachnowski, S. (2012). Special delivery: An analysis of mHealth in maternal and newborn health programs and their outcomes around the world. *Maternal and Child Health Journal, 16*(5), 1092–1101.

The Economist. (2014, April 5). The rise of the cheap smartphone. *The Economist.* Retrieved from http://www.economist.com/news/business/21600134-smartphones-reach-masses-host-vendors-are-eager-serve-them-rise-cheap. Accessed 5 Jan 2017.

Thondoo, M., Strachan, D. L., Nakirunda, M., Ndima, S., Muiambo, A., Källander, K., ...InSCALE Study Group (2015). Potential roles of Mhealth for community health workers: Formative research with end users in Uganda and Mozambique. *JMIR mHealth and uHealth, 3*(3).

Timm, T. (2014, May 3). Technology law will soon be reshaped by people who don't use email. *The Guardian.* Retrieved from theguardian.com/commentisfree/2014/may/03/technology-law-us-supreme-court-internet-nsa. Accessed 9 Jan 2017.

Tomlinson, M., Solomon, W., Singh, Y., Doherty, T., Chopra, M., Ijumba, P., ...Jackson, D. (2009). The use of mobile phones as a data collection tool: A report from a household survey in South Africa. *BMC Medical Informatics and Decision Making, 9*(1), 51.

Tomlinson, M., Rotheram-Borus, M. J., Swartz, L., & Tsai, A. C. (2013). Scaling up mHealth: Where is the evidence? *PLoS Med, 10*(2), e1001382.

Umali, E., McCool, J., & Whittaker, R. (2016). Possibilities and expectations for mHealth in the Pacific Islands: Insights from key informants. *JMIR mHealth and uHealth, 4*(1).

van Heerden, A., Tomlinson, M., & Swartz, L. (2012). Point of care in your pocket: A research agenda for the field of m-health. *Bulletin of the World Health Organization, 90*(5), 393–394.

Waugaman, A. (2016). *From principle to practice: Implementing the principles for digital development. Perspectives and Recommendations from the Practitioner Community.* Washington, DC: The Principles for Digital Development Working Group, 1–76. Retrieved from http://www.unicefstories.org/wp-content/uploads/2013/08/From_Principle_to_Practice.pdf.

Whittaker, R., Merry, S., Dorey, E., & Maddison, R. (2012). A development and evaluation process for mHealth interventions: Examples from New Zealand. *Journal of Health Communication, 17*(sup1), 11–21.

World Bank (2011, June 21). World Bank supports cross-border energy cooperation between India and Nepal. [Press release]. *World Bank.* Retrieved from http://www.worldbank.org/en/news/press-release/2011/06/21/world-bank-supports-cross-border-energy-cooperation-between-india-and-nepal. Accessed 4 Jan 2017.

World Bank (2016a). *World Bank open data: Mobile cellular subscriptions (per 100 people).* Retrieved from http://data.worldbank.org/indicator/IT.CEL.SETS.P2 . Accessed 5 Jan 2017.

World Bank (2016b). *World Bank open data: Access to electricity (% of population).* Retrieved from http://data.worldbank.org/indicator/EG.ELC.ACCS.ZS. Accessed 5 Jan 2017.

World Health Organization (2016). *Global diffusion of eHealth: Making universal health coverage achievable. Report of the third global survey on eHealth.* Geneva: World Health Organization. Retrieved from http://who.int/goe/publications/global_diffusion/en/. Accessed 7 Jan 2017.

Zurovac, D., Sudoi, R. K., Akhwale, W. S., Ndiritu, M., Hamer, D. H., Rowe, A. K., et al. (2011). The effect of mobile phone text-message reminders on Kenyan health workers' adherence to malaria treatment guidelines: A cluster randomised trial. *The Lancet, 378*(9793), 795–803.

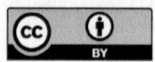

Chapter 4
The Use of Mobile Phones in Rural Javanese Villages: Knowledge Production and Information Exchange Among Poor Women with Diabetes

Dyah Pitaloka

Abstract Previous studies have found mHealth-based smartphone applications are promising tools to help improve diabetes management and self-care. However, rural populations are often not smartphone-equipped and therefore cannot access diabetes management apps. Guided by a culture-centered approach, this chapter describes an ethnographic study of health behaviors among women in two Javanese villages. In-depth interviews were conducted with 30 female participants in Central Java, Indonesia. Grounded theory was adopted for data analysis. This study sought to unearth the existing modes of communication and it was found that—in conversation with *mantri* (a male health practitioner)—the participants developed alternative modes of mHealth communication based on SMS. The sending and receiving of diabetes-related SMS became embedded in the women's daily lives and enabled them to navigate their health routines as people living with diabetes.

Keywords Diabetes · Self-management · mHealth · Culture-centered approach Rural Javanese women · Indonesia

4.1 Introduction

According to one estimate, the number of SIM card subscriptions in Indonesia at January 2016 was 326.3 million (We Are Social, 2016). Given that the total population of Indonesia numbers around 255 million individuals (Indonesia Population Census, 2010) with the adult population estimated at 150 million, this means many people have more than one device and/or SIM cards. It also indicates that large numbers of the poor now have mobile phones. Indeed, over the past decade, lower service prices have attracted new consumer segments to enter the market. Prepaid Internet packages for smartphones range from US$ 0.50 a day to $2.50 a month

D. Pitaloka (✉)
Department of Indonesian Studies, University of Sydney, Sydney, Australia
e-mail: dyah.pitaloka@sydney.edu.au

© Asian Development Bank 2018
E. Baulch et al. (eds.), *mHealth Innovation in Asia*, Mobile Communication in Asia:
Local Insights, Global Implications, https://doi.org/10.1007/978-94-024-1251-2_4

(freedom-net Indonesia, 2015). This low service price allowed new consumer segments with limited spending capacity to enter the market.

For rural people, a prepaid tariff (*prabayar*)—commonly known as buying "*pulsa*" (prepaid mobile phones minutes)—is the most common mode of connecting to mobile networks. *Pulsa* is sold in the market, on the street and in grocery shops in electronic form or as vouchers. In most cities, *pulsa* vendors are open 24 hour and apply only a small extra charge for their service. *Pulsa* can also be purchased via ATMs, e-banking, and 24-hour convenience stores without extra charge. In villages, people usually go to the market to buy *pulsa* or to their neighbor who becomes an individual *pulsa* reseller.

The number of people suffering from diabetes is rising globally and impoverished rural populations are at higher risk of poor self-management and complications associated with the illness (Banerjee, Rathod, Konda, & Bhawalkar, 2014; Hsu et al., 2012; Pujilestari, Ng, Hakimi, & Eriksson, 2014; Utz et al., 2008). 2013 data from RISKEDAS indicate that 10 million people have been diagnosed with diabetes in Indonesia, with roughly equal figures for adult diabetes prevalence in rural and urban areas (7 and 6.8%, respectively). This puts Indonesia among the top five countries for diabetes prevalence (WHO, 2016) with most cases recorded on the island of Java. More than 70% of the cases were undiagnosed and women are reported as more susceptible than men.

Previous studies have found mHealth-based smartphone applications are promising tools to help improve diabetes management and self-care (Cui, Wu, Mao, Wang, & Nie, 2016; Shah & Garg, 2015). For instance, mobile phone interventions for people with diabetes can improve healthcare outcomes by facilitating an individual's ability to control, monitor, and measure blood sugar level and thereby adopt healthier behaviors (Kitsiou, Pare, Jaana, & Gerber, 2017; Krishna & Boren, 2008). Indeed patients' adherence to self-management regimes is recognized as a marker of success for mHealth intervention. However, rural populations are often not smartphone-equipped and therefore cannot access diabetes management apps.

This study adopts the culture-centered approach (Dutta, 2008, 2011) to enquire into the role of local women's organizations and networks in encouraging rural women's use of mobile phones for sharing and disseminating information about health and sugar disease. Central to the culture-centered approach is that health communication involves "the negotiation of shared meanings embedded in socially constructed identities, relationships, social norms, and structures" (Dutta, 2008: 55). Therefore, the main target of diabetes communication interventions is culture.

Javanese women have been perceived as being tied to three domestic areas: kitchen, bedroom, and washing area (well). Studies conducted on Javanese women (Manderson, 1983; Sears, 1996; Sullivan, 1983, 1994; Wolf, 1994) suggested that due to their long working hours, women have less time than men to socialize and be involved in religious activities. However, this study found that women are actively engaged in both social and religious activities including women's rotating credit associations or saving-and-loan activities (*arisan*) and Qur'an recitation groups (*pengajian*), both of which serve as important forms for the promotion of women's health and well-being.

Eight months of ethnographic fieldwork were conducted in two villages located about 1 hour south of Magelang municipality in the Central Java province. This study was part of my larger study of women, culture, and diabetes in Java. Through a close contact with a local male health provider (*mantri* in Indonesian), I managed to conduct observations and in-depth interviews with 30 women from two villages. Being familiar with the district and as a fluent speaker of the Javanese language, I managed to connect with my participants and was invited to their houses to observe their everyday activities and to experience the challenges they faced. I also attended recitations and *arisan* to understand the interactions among rural women in the villages.

4.2   Traditional Gender Roles in Rural Java and Women's Autonomy

My quest to understand how poor rural women manage diabetes took me to a late afternoon conversation with *mantri* (local male health provider) with whom I have been collaborating for this research. He discussed his concerns about the increasing number of people, especially women, suffering diabetes in the villages. Most of the time his patients had to be hospitalized because they do not know about the severity of the disease and how to monitor their blood sugar level. According to *mantri*, rural women work very hard to support their families and "because of their hard life, these women get so tough. They won't let anything interrupt their routines, including illness. Therefore, it requires extra patience to talk to them about their health issues."

Traditional gender roles in rural areas in Java assigned women with managerial positions both in domestic and public (societal) spheres. Rural women in both the *Kembangarum*[1] and *Selojajar*[1] villages investigated in this study mostly work as petty traders. In 2014, poor rural villagers in Central Java were estimated to earn between US$20 and 40/month (BPS Jateng, 2014). Therefore, the villagers live on less than US$2/day and must balance their everyday needs with the social costs required to maintain harmonious interactions within the village. The work and the money they earned gave these rural women a sense of self-reliance and of space to negotiate their personal needs. For example, Wani (all participant names have been replaced with pseudonyms) said:

> Having a job, earning my own money, I can 'move' myself around a little bit (*Neknyambut damel, nyekel arta piyambak, kula saged 'obah' - obah* or move literary means 'a more flexible condition that allows someone to make a decision amidst his/her limited resources).

Participants expressed that it is important for them to keep working and to earn their own money, because by having their own income, these women could:

---

[1]Pseudonyms used.

(1) participate more in *arisan*, (2) fulfill personal needs (such as seeing a doctor or *mantri*, purchasing medication, buying a mobile phone, or topping up phone credit), (3) give pocket money to their children or grandchildren, and (4) donate to their neighbors and social events in the villages.

The day starts at 4 am every morning for many of these women. After performing early morning prayers, those who sell traditional snacks such as banana and/or vegetable fritters must have all the food ready by 6 am. They then must complete all chores and be ready to go to the market by 7.30 am. None of them questioned this division of labor, which saw them responsible for both household duties and working outside of the home. During interview, Parti said:

> "To make sure that the house is clean and the food for my family is ready before I go to the market is important to me. I feel guilty if I wake up late and leave the house in a messy condition" [Javanese would say *mboten ilok* (taboo)].

None of the women lamented their health condition or complained about having to work to support their family. Some of them walk as far as 15 km to the market while carrying a 30 kg basket filled with merchandise. Others take public transportation to do the trading in the next village. They usually return home at around 5 pm before *magrib* (after sunset) the fourth of five formal daily prayers for Muslims, so they can join the mass prayer in the mosque with other villagers.

Their sense of self-reliance and the ability to perform domestic responsibilities and maintain multiple roles within the household and the community is of central importance to these women. As petty traders, the women do not earn big money. But they do earn a degree of economic autonomy and an ability to manage and control household spending.

I observed that by being petty traders, these women attain a strong sense of self-reliance and bargaining power to take decisions regarding both household matters and social affairs in the village more broadly. The women believe that the ability to perform daily activities represents a core component of being a good Javanese woman—self-reliant, strong, an effective manager of the household, makes household financial decisions autonomously, and with the power to manage social networks (Geertz, 1961; Jay, 1969; Koentjaraningrat, 1967; Pitaloka, 2014; Pitaloka & Hsieh, 2015). Many of these women display a high degree of discipline in their management of finances. While showing me an old wooden box full of labeled envelopes, Restu explained her strategy for managing the family's limited income:

> I'm poor, so I must manage the money we earned each day. This is to buy groceries, rice, washing soap, shampoo. This is for my youngest son's school fee, this is for the mosque, and this is for other social events. These social events always give me headache, but it's important. This one envelope is actually for my personal needs, but it also serves as a secure funding for me. I use the money from this envelope to buy my medicines or *pulsa*, but if I received too many social events invitations, I will use it to cover the social events first.

4.3   Mobile Phone and Health Needs Among Rural Village Women

Understanding how these women perceive and negotiate their multiple roles is crucial to grasping existing mHealth practices. Using the culture-centered approach, this study located the cultural factors that influenced—and were influenced by—the everyday narratives of health and well-being experienced by these rural Javanese women. For instance, Tuti's description of her mobile phone use demonstrated the organic emergence of personal mHealth behaviors:

> This is a cheap phone. I got it from the market. My son asked me to get one so he can contact me if something urgent happens. I rarely use it...well, mostly for receiving calls. Sometimes, I use it to call Pak[2] *mantri* to have a health check, or to order some stuffs from the city. Pak *mantri* send me texts and calls to make sure that I take my medicines and attend the monthly health meeting at his house. He and his wife are very nice to me.

Some rural women in this study purchased mobile phones with money saved through arisan saving-and-loan scheme, while others use their own savings to purchase cheap mobile phones at the market. Some rural women in these villages are still practicing a traditional saving method by keeping their money inside a small envelope or in a wooden box, which they keep in a safe place at home. Some of the older women participants were bought mobile phones by their children. As mentioned, the phones enabled them to stay connected with their family members (i.e., husband, children, and grandchildren), fellow traders, friends, and also with *mantri*.

While the women perceived doctors as socially higher than them, and therefore they feel *sungkan* (Javanese respectful behavior that means feeling of shame without the feeling of doing something wrong) to call or text them, they perceived *mantri* as part of their family. They felt they could contact *mantri* whenever they needed his help or advice. "I usually visit my patients one by one...riding this motorbike, going around the villages," *mantri* explained. Living in the same neighborhood as the women, *mantri* and his family are considered as kin. Regardless of their resource-poor conditions, these women highly appreciated the "inner peace" (*ketenangan batin*) that a mobile phone brought to their life. Samsiah said:

> I don't really need a mobile phone, but one day I was very sick. I don't know why, but I felt weak and suddenly collapsed. When I woke up, I was already in the hospital. *Pak mantri* told me, 'Alhamdulillah (Thank God) my wife was already at your door when your sister cried out for help.' After I recovered, my son got me a used phone...He told me, '*Mak* (mom), just in case. *Pak mantri* can check on you. If you refuse [to take the phone], I won't let you go to the market again' Well, it's hard for me to use it at first, but I feel *ayem* (peace). I can work and my son won't have to worry about me.

---

[2]*Pak* is an abbreviation of *Bapak*, originally meaning 'father' but nowadays used to respectfully address an adult male.

Rural women of low education and socioeconomic status are important actors in the informal sector (as market traders, factory workers, and housemaids) of the economy, significant providers within their families (Kusujiarti, 1997; Tickamyer & Kusujiarti, 2012; Wolf, 1994), and overrepresented in various indices of poor health. Many of the women lack medical knowledge of diabetes symptoms, but have developed their own language to articulate their experience of living with diabetes. They perceive diabetes as less severe than cancer, asthma, heart disease, and skin problems because their diabetes was asymptomatic and their condition is relatively stable. As they say, they are "not stranded in bed" and are able to perform everyday duties (Pitaloka, 2014). When their blood sugar level increases, these women would express it as "they do not feel well" or "too much in mind" (*kakehan pikiran*).

These vernacular understandings of the causes and symptoms of diabetes grow up in context of several gaps left by top-down approaches to health care and the exclusion of much of the rural population from web connectivity, increasingly central to the ability to access professional medical information. Currently, Indonesian health system still focuses more on battling infectious diseases such as malaria, tuberculosis, diarrhea, and dengue fever. Resources have not been allocated proportionally to the larger and increasingly threatening burden of chronic noncommunicable diseases such as heart diseases, stroke, diabetes, cancer, and hypertension (Ng et al., 2006). A yawning gap also exists between the promise of a technologically determined health utopia and the reality of actual uses and access to such technologies among poor and rural populations.

The rapid growth of mobile telephony is often held to create an opportunity for the emergence of mHealth—the use of mobile communication devices for health services and information, in improving the access and quality of health services, and overall health outcomes in many parts of the world, including facilitating diabetes self-management (Chib, 2010; Chib & Chen, 2011; Chigona, Nyemba-Mudenda, & Metfula, 2013; Kratzke, Wilson, & Vilchis, 2013; Klasnja & Pratt, 2012; Kreps & Neuhaser, 2010; Soegijoko, 2009). In Indonesia, mHealth designers have produced apps such as *Dokter Diabetes* and *Xanesha Diabetic Analytic Console* to encourage individuals with diabetes to self-manage their illness. A few mHealth apps developed by foreign companies were also available such as *Diabetes:M* by Sirma Medical Systems, the Dario app by Dario Health, *OnTrack Diabetes* and *BlueStar Diabetes*.

The enthusiastic development of health self-management apps so often proceeds with disregard for the technical, socioeconomic, and cultural barriers that stand in the way of poor, rural, and marginalized people using them (Kaplan, 2006). In Indonesia, the available diabetes mHealth applications can only be accessed through Android and iOS smartphones—use of which is largely restricted to middle and upper social economic groups. The use of mix languages (English and Indonesian) requires users to understand the terms used by the providers, such as "check-up record" and "diabetes risk". In addition, these applications require patients to understand their diabetic condition, especially their blood sugar level and the medication regime they have taken. Such mHealth interventions, then, reflect approaches to health promotion have largely focused on public individual cognitive determinants that often neglect the social structure and cultural aspects that surrounds those individuals (Green, Richard, & Potvin, 1996; Patrick, Intille, & Zabinski, 2005; Sallis & Owen, 2002).

Moreover, issues of connectivity and cost also restrict many rural dwellers' access to the Internet. For example, prepaid mobile phone users in Indonesia must have a minimum data plan which varies between Rp 10,000 to unlimited in order to be able to access the Internet. The women in this study spend between Rp 10,000 and Rp 20,000 per month to keep their number. This urban-rural inequality in Internet access (Indonesian national socioeconomic survey/Susenas 2010–2012; Sujarwoto & Tampubolon, 2016) excludes the poor from accessing health-related information. As health information increasingly circulates online, and health interventions are linked to costly devices and English proficiency, many rural poor can be "rendered voiceless through inaccess to this communication platforms where policies are debated, implemented, and evaluated" (Dutta, 2008, p. 149).

4.4   Culture and Rural Women's Use of Mobile Phones

As petty traders and income earners, these rural women do not rely on their husbands' wages to fulfill their personal needs. Nor do those who no longer have a husband (by death or divorce) rely on their children's support for their living. One of them said, "As parents, we should be the one to help our children, not the one to burden them." This behavior is guided by the Javanese sense of "*pekewuh*" (ashamed in the presence of one's better), a feeling induced by asking your husband or children for a favor. The maintenance of harmony, order, and self-mastery are key tenets of Javanese social work (Immajati, 1996; Mulder, 1996; Pitaloka, 2014), and this context is crucial to understanding rural women's uses of mobile phones.

Cheap mobile phones are sold at the local phone shop or at the market with the price for between Rp 150,000 ($15) and Rp 250,000 ($25). Such phones provide basic mobile phone calling and SMS services that according to these women, "is enough" (*cukup*) and "appropriate" (*cocok, pas*). The notion of *cukup* and *pas* represent the Javanese cultural notions of appreciation and sincere acceptance that forbid them from being greedy. Siti said:

> Since I got diabetes, my children have been asking me to buy a phone so they can check on my condition. I feel reluctant, because I could not use the household money just to buy a mobile phone. I refused when my children want to get me one, because I know they also have a hard life. I got this one when I got the *arisan* money. Just a cheap one…as long as my children can contact me, it's enough.

Cukup reflects a sense of self-control that implies women's ability to control complex interactions within the self (at a personal level) and with others (at a social level). Women are constantly reminded to carefully manage money in order to support basic household needs and to be able to perform social obligations in the village (e.g., contribute appropriate *sumbangan* (gifts) to other villagers at lifecycle rituals).

Women in this study confirmed that they use their mobile phones mostly for making and receiving a call. They would respond to a text message, only when someone texted them first. Calling is much easier for these women, especially the older ones. This finding echoes the LIRNEasia qualitative demand-side study 'Teleuse at the Bottom of the Pyramid 4' (2011) which found that 89% of rural poor women in Java used their mobile phones mostly for making a voice call (see Fig. 4.1).

Women in this study explained that having a mobile phone means extra spending, and they are aware that this spending must not interfere with their household needs. Tasriyah said "If I need to top up my phone credit, I don't buy too much. As long as it's enough to call my children and *Pak mantri*. I must carefully manage my money." All women in this study used prepaid since it enabled them to control their spending. As daily wage earners, these women are aware that their main concern is their family. Anti said:

> My daughter got me this phone to learn my whereabouts. I rarely make a call. I will top up my credit if I have spare money, if not then wait until I get money. Sometimes, I forgot [to buy pulsa] and I have to buy a new number [because the subscription expires when you do not recharge]. If my son has extra money, sometimes he buys me Rp 20,000 ($2) and it lasts for 2 to 3 weeks. I don't want to trouble my kids. I never spend much.

Anti's statement echoes the LIRNEasia (2011) data which indicates that bottom of pyramid mobile users with irregular income use a prepaid card to limit their phone credit spending (see Fig. 4.2).

In addition, this study found that a sense of *pekewuh* (feeling of reluctant or uncomfortable from doing something that is considered as culturally inappropriate) guided women's use of mobile phones. These women do not want to be preoc-

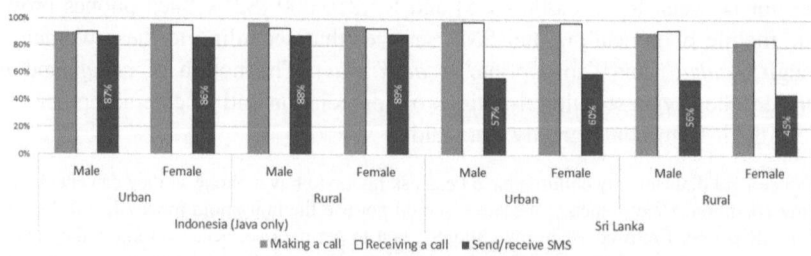

Fig. 4.1 Mobile phone use by bottom of pyramid mobile owners (LIRNEasia, 2011)

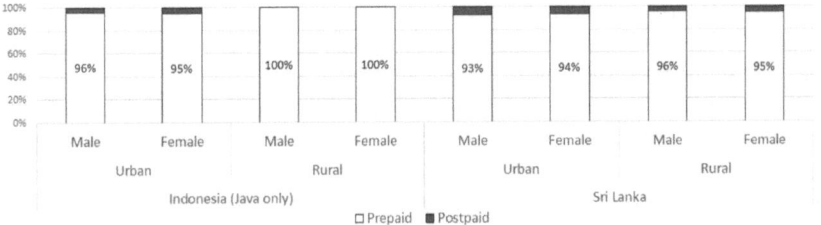

Fig. 4.2 Prepaid versus Postpaid use by bottom of pyramid mobile owners (LIRNEasia, 2011)

cupied with their phones when they are at home. Some of these women share the house and kitchen with their children's family. To maintain harmonious life, one of them said, "*Kudu njogo, ngerti wong liyo*," which can be translated as considering and appreciating others (*tepa selira*). They used their phones in their 'private domains' e.g. at the market, at *arisan* or at *pengajian*. Javanese society perceives women as in control at the marketplace (Brenner, 1998) hence the women considered it appropriate to act as they chose in this domain.

4.5   Text Message as an Alternative Communicative Space

With such limited material resources, exchanging health-related text messages is an organic community activity that encourages these rural women to participate in the health-seeking process as well as knowledge production. *Mantri* plays a vital role as an initiator. In most villages, in Indonesia, *mantri* plays an important role in providing health-related support and educating rural people about health (Ferzacca, 1996; Geertz, 1961; Harper & Amrith, 2014). When I asked him why he thinks that texting could be the solution, *mantri* said:

> Actually, they have mobile phones, but they don't use it. If I don't call them, they won't call me. If I don't remind them 'don't forget to have your blood sugar check' 'don't forget to drink your medication'…well…they will remain quiet. Then before I know it, their son or family member is calling me because my patient is unconscious. They could've use their phones to ask me: 'why do I have such and such a problem' 'what do I do when I have such and such a symptom', so I can help them before it's too late'. But then, the problem is, they don't really know what to ask, right?

Above, I have discussed how limited material resources excluded these poor rural women from accessing and experiencing health and health care. The enthusiastic development of mHealth apps may well serve generously resourced urban communities in Indonesia, but can fail to reach community members like the women in this study. The texting activities I have described above address the local contexts that framed Javanese health beliefs and the complexity of the rural women's needs and priorities. They also provide an alternative communicative space for these rural women to experience health and maintain their well-being.

As a progressive disease, type 2 diabetes may cause complications and disability over time. The women in this study articulated their health condition by using these words: *semangat* (spirit or energy) which symbolizes health, and *lemes* (weak) or *loyo* (exhausted) which symbolizes illness (Ferzacca, 2001; Pitaloka, 2014). These women believed that diabetes is caused by hard thoughts and a restless mind. Therefore, balancing ones' inner peace (*ati tentrem*) with outer/physical health (*awak penak*) is perceived to be the main key to health. Participating in informal local organizations, such as *arisan* and *pengajian* Quran is an occasion to relax and to get-together with other women in the village. Sarni, for example, expressed her participation in recitation as:

> All of these burdens and hard thoughts are gone. I tried to come to recitation, at least once a month to recharge myself. When I recite Quran together, I feel peace and calm. *Gusti* (God) always listens to our prayer, right? The leader [of the recitation] is also very nice and funny. The discussion is light, so I can understand [the context and application of the *surah* (chapter) being recited].

Mantri's wife also participated in these local women's organizations. In addition, she was also a volunteer at *posyandu* (community health and nutrition integrated service center)—a center which is run by the community and provides services, such as Family Planning, Mother and Child Health, Nutrition (growth monitoring, supplemental feeding, vitamin and mineral supplementation, and nutrition education), Immunization, and Diarrhea Disease Control (Anwar, Khomsan, Sukandar, Riyadi, & Mudjajanto, 2010).

Facilitating Self-help: With the help of his wife Dwi and two women volunteers Erna and Tuti, *mantri* began to initiate texting activities back in 2012. His simple aim was to text those villagers that he could not visit due to his schedule to encourage them to be actively involved in their personal healthcare. He also wished to encourage his diabetic patients to participate in taking care of their own health as well as their friends'. When I asked *mantri* why he focused his efforts so much on women, he said:

> Women in these villages are very self-reliant and they take care of everything. They attended *arisan, pengajian*, and volunteering to hold *Posyandu* meeting each month. They prepare the food and work to earn money to support the family. And most importantly, my diabetic patients are mostly women…

Mantri relies on SMS to communicate with the women because it is cheaper than calling, the user does not need to download separate application—texting comes as a basic application with the mobile phone, and because texting does not require the women to respond immediately. During the first year, *mantri* sent SMS mostly to remind his patients about *posyandu* activities and free monthly blood sugar check sessions. When I came to *mantri*'s house to talk to him about this texting activity, he had just sent an SMS to his patient to remind her to have blood sugar check in the coming week,

> Please don't think too hard, *Bu* [Mrs] Sih. Calm your mind. Don't forget the free blood sugar check on Thursday.

A few minutes later, he received a phone call. *Mantri* told me, smiling, "I texted my patient and she asked her son to call me and asked if she needs to do a test this month because her glucose was 250 last month and she feels fine." Although this woman did not reply to *mantri*'s SMS in person, the call shows that she engages with the message and the communication activity. Erna, one of the posyandu volunteers and *arisan* coordinator who joined us that afternoon told me:

> Now, I can use my phone to send health information to my friends. I don't use it for casual chatting with friends, I use it when there's important issue we can help each other, by reminding each other.

When I asked Erna what kind of information she and the other women discussed, she said

> Usually about…mmm…free blood sugar check session, or if there's an information session at *Pak mantri*'s house. I myself have diabetes for 5 years, and my two kids are still very small. I'm stupid and poor, but giving information to my friends and getting advice on keeping my physical condition fresh (*seger* = *sehat* = healthy) is good.

Tuti, the other volunteer, confirmed what Erna said about "reminding each other." In fact, *arisan* and *pengajian*, as well as *posyandu*, are forms of rural women's self-help that provide assistance in emergencies such as accidents, deaths, and illnesses. Texting opens up opportunities for these rural women to communicate about their condition, like text that *mantri* received after we broke the fast one evening: *Niki kula kok awake adem kabeh ndrodog, pripun pak?* (I feel cold and trembly, what should I do?). Without further due, *mantri* took his motorcycle and went to this woman's house. I rode with Dwi. It turned out that this woman did not take her early breakfast properly and experience a hypoglycemic condition—low blood sugar.

Negotiating Knowledge: Advice, as Erna said, is a form of "knowledge negotiation" which refers to women's active participation and involvement in knowledge production via texting. Rather than acting as users, *mantri* and these rural women act as the cocreators of knowledge in their texting. Diabetes knowledge, as promoted by doctors, focused on three things: Food intake management, regular consumption of medication, and exercise. This model of self-management detached these women from their everyday values. As a top-down form of intervention, this knowledge does not take into account the sociocultural, religious, and economic aspects that framed these rural women's concept of health, the dynamic of interactions between the villagers, and Javanese traditional concept of gender roles.

Health, in these women's perceptions lies within their heart and mind. Marni explains that:

> As long as your mind is calm, you'll feel that you're healthier. Fasting, attending Qur'an recitation, helps ease your mind.

I had a chance to observe the daily activity of one of the older participants, Prapti, who told me:

> I asked pak mantri if people with sugar disease can fast or not?

She continued

> He said I can, as long I don't forget to take my medicines. I just texted my friend: you should fast. I don't feel weak and I can recite Qur'an till late at night.

On another occasion, I went to meet a mother and daughter who both had diabetes. When I came to Lis's (the mother's) house, she told me that her daughter Nani's blood sugar level is constantly high and she was certain that her daughter's heavy thoughts triggered this condition. During the interview, Lis told me that she just asked her youngest daughter to text Nani using her mobile phone: *Ora kejeron mikir. Ayem, sumeleh gusti kaya Ibuk, ben gulomu medhun* (don't think too much. Stay calm and surrender to God and, like me, your glucose level will go down). With her eye condition, Lis could not read small letters clearly.

Managing food intake/diet is a concept that some of these rural women find hard to negotiate. With limited income, these women do not have many choices. For them, food should sustain their physical strength in order to work all day. In addition, because earning money is difficult, these women never throw away leftover rice. *Mantri*'s wife told me that she received a text from one woman who said that since she consumed *sega wadhang* (cold leftover rice), her glucose level becomes stable. I asked *mantri*'s wife, "Is it true?" and Dwi said, "Most women here believed that cold leftover rice cures diabetes, but I always tell them that they can eat *sega wadhang*, but don't forget to have some vegetables in their meal for nutrition."

Alternative medicine is another topic that these women talk about when texting. Traditional home remedies known as *jamu* are very popular among rural people. They perceived *jamu* as the first solution to illness and *jamu* is widely consumed to maintain physical fitness. Abundant resources of herbal plantations are available across the villages, such as ginger, turmeric, betel leaf, etc. I noted that one of the reasons why some rural women choose to incorporate alternative medicines such as traditional herbal drinks or *jamu* in their diabetes management was to find a treatment that is appropriate (*cocok*) to their financial condition (Pitaloka, 2014). During one *arisan* meeting, these women discussed *jamu* and Erna told me that she received many texts about diabetes *jamu* recipes, such as soursop leaf drink, bitter gourd drink, and turmeric drinks.

Fostering Women's Consciousness about Health: A restless heart and heavy thoughts are believed to be the cause of diabetes. While managing inner peace becomes the women's main attention, *mantri*'s role is to inform the women about the importance of maintaining their blood sugar level. Texting encourages these women to become more conscious about their health. In one of the recitation meetings that I attended, the women discussed why the Qur'an had to say with respect to health. Preaching in Javanese, the leader of the recitation wrapped up the session that night with this message:

> Nothing is worse than someone who is overeating – filling her stomach with food that exceeds its capacity. If you eat, do eat to make your body strong and straight (*tegak*). But remember, you should allow 1/3 of your stomach for food, 1/3 for drinks, and 1/3 for breath.

This closing provoked the women to discuss their eating habits. After the recitation, Warni invited me to her house to break the fast. She came to the recitation with her daughter who lives in a different village. That night her daughter went back straight away since her infant had a slight fever. While preparing the food, Warni talked about the reason she keeps working and about her daughter who is always concerned about Warni's health condition. Since she lives in a different village, Warni's daughter used a mobile phone to check on her mother's condition. She told me, "*Niki, nembe mawon nyambel kok anake malah sms, ngeten niki to…*" (see, I just finished making sambal and my daughter had already texted me): *Mak, maeme dijogo* (watch your meal mom). Laughing, Warni said, "*Kula niki mung wong ra nduwe, mangan sega sambel. Saka pasar ngelih....eh, ora entuk mangan akeh*" (I'm poor and I only eat sambal and rice. I feel hungry coming home from the market and I can't eat a bigger portion).

The concept of eating for Warni was not about the variety of food on the plate, the price, or how healthy the food is. Eating was about the ability to enjoy food no matter how simple it is. For her, the simple dish of warm rice and sambal (Javanese chili with shrimp paste aroma) brings a joyful feeling. She could have finished two plates of rice for herself, especially when she comes home from work tired and hungry. A glass of sweet hot tea would accompany her meal. Of course, this diet does not fit the concept of healthy eating for diabetes management but rice and sambal are a source of happiness for Marni—an emotional condition that eases other burdens in life. However, that night Marni only had a half plate of rice, sambal, and three deep-fried *tempe* (soya bean cake).

The sermon also promoted *mantri*'s wife to send texts to two *posyandu* women volunteers who had been working with her for years and had diabetes, highlighting how the circulation of health information, texting and attendance, and discussions at recitation meetings are all interrelated parts of a whole way of life.

> Don't forget to do your [noon] prayer. Eat properly, don't eat too much to stay healthy. Amiin.

The other topic that the women discussed was personal hygiene. After the *posyandu* session, one woman told *mantri* that she prefers to go barefoot because wearing shoes made her feel uncomfortable. She believed herself not to be at risk of developing infection from a wound, stating that she only suffered dry diabetes. *Mantri* responded, "It's better to be careful. Wearing footwear is good for your cleanliness and health." In an interview with Sri, who grows turmeric and other herbs, I asked "Why don't you wear footwear?" Sri responded:

> We're just villagers, I myself also love walking around barefoot, but I feel bad now because *Bu mantri* said in her text: *kebersihan niku bagian dari iman* (cleanliness is part of faith).

Wearing footwear outside the house to prevent any cuts or wounds is a key tenet of maintaining diabetic health because diabetics are at a high risk of cuts or wounds becoming infected. Indeed, when one of the women's family members had to undergo amputation due to infection, *mantri* sent a text message to the two volunteers Erna and Tuti so they could share the news with others:

> *Ampun lali ngagem sandal nek medhal ben mboten keno beling nopo paku sing saged damel infeksi* (don't forget to wear footwear if you're doing activities outside the house, so your feet won't get slashed and wounded in ways that may cause infection).

The other topic that engaged these rural women in texting was managing their food intake at community social events. One text that *mantri* received was:

> What should I eat if I have to attend a wedding or *slametan* (Javanese ritual meal)?

For rural Javanese, everyday life from birth to death revolves around ceremonies and social celebrations and these events always involve feasting. Participating in social events like *slametan* is very important for the rural people. Moreover, women are responsible for preparing food for such events and this presents a challenge for diabetics. One woman who used to help with cooking sent a message to Tuti: *Nek ora diicipi wedi ra enak, ning meh kabeh legi. Piye yo?* (if I don't taste the food, I'm afraid that the taste is not quite right, but almost all are sweet, what should I do?). Bu *mantri* who listened to this story from Tuti sent a text message: *Ngicipi nek sakjumput/saksesepan mboten nopo2, ampun sak enthong* (tasting, if it's a pinch/a sip is ok, but don't take a large soup spoon).

In my travels to the local market, I came across a drink called *tetes*—a thick red sugary syrup that is popular among the locals because of its refreshing taste, electric pink color, and cheap price. People usually mix *tetes* with water and ice to make *es tetes*—an irresistibly refreshing drink for a hot day at the market. When I met *mantri* later that evening, he told me that some of the women had been enquiring about the health effects of the food they consume daily, including *tetes*. For example, one of his patients texted him to ask: *Nopo tetes saged nginggilaken gendis?* (Could *tetes* drink increase my blood sugar?). When I interviewed this woman, Darni, she explained that her glucose level was constantly high and she wanted to know whether her love for *tetes* caused this problem, "If you're poor, it's a refreshing drink that poor people can afford, because it's cheap. I can drink two glasses especially during a long hot day at the market." *Mantri* responded to Darni's text with simple suggestion:

> Please try to drink water. It's better not to overconsume anything. Please try to reduce your *tetes* consumption.

Knowing that these women may not be aware of the dangers of overconsuming sugar, *mantri* raised issue at the monthly health information session. At that time, there were at least 15 women with diabetes who joined both *arisan* and *pengajian* group and five others who only joined *pengajian*. Tuti told me, "*Mboten gampang le ngandani, wong kula mawon remen tetes kok*" (It's not easy to tell the women what to do, I personally also like *tetes*). If someone asked her about it, she forwarded *mantri*'s SMS:

Water is good for your health. It's refreshing and cheap.

It seems that "cheap" is the key word in this SMS because *mantri* received a good response to it including short texts such as "*leres*" (true), "*sae njih*?" (oh, it's good?!), to longer questions: "is just ordinary boiled water OK or bottled water?" "I can't quit drinking coffee, is it bad?"

4.6 Conclusion

This study highlights the value of organic texting activity among the rural women participants as a form of continuous reflection upon their health. The positive effects of using SMS cannot just be attributed to technological affordance, which is where the emphasis of mHealth discourse can often lie. It can also be attributed to the dynamic interplay of culture—the shared values, practices, and meanings that are negotiated in communities—and structure, understood as the system that enables or constraints these women's access to resources.

On one hand, texting provides an alternative communication space for these women to discuss possible solutions to their health problems while reflecting their cultural beliefs. The advice that these women receive from each other and from *mantri* can be seen as a form of "knowledge negotiation"—which refers to women's active participation and involvement in knowledge production via texting. Contrary to the dominant mHealth approach in which app providers act as knowledge generators and mobile phone subscribers as users, *mantri* and these rural women act as cocreators of knowledge related to their health. On the other hand, texting provides a communicative space for these women to develop peer support and the capacity for agency and autonomy. In the process of cocreating knowledge, women and *mantri* negotiate living with diabetes in the context of everyday life. Despite their poverty, these women still hold considerable power in the management of both domestic and public affairs in the villages. Thus, the SMS exchanges that occur between them and *mantri* reflect their need to balance these roles and maintain harmonious social interactions.

Global discourses around diabetes management frame the failure of patients' diabetes management as related to individual action or inaction (Aikins, Boyton, & Atanga, 2010; McKee, Clarke, Kmetic, & Reading, 2009; Parry, Peel, Douglas, & Lawton, 2006). This suggests that poor health occurs because individuals are unable or unwilling to heed preventive messages or recommended treatment actions

(Airhihenbuwa, Ford, & Iwenlunmor, 2014). Being poor and having diabetes, the women in this study constantly negotiated their personal needs (including their health needs) with those of their family and community. As a result, their health-seeking behaviors must be compatible with the other elements of life, i.e., a good "fit" (*cocok*) (Pitaloka, 2014).

From a culture-centered approach, texting is woven into these women's experience of diabetes and how they negotiate their health-seeking behaviors. The messages are not centralized or controlled by one person. Instead, messages flow from SMS to discussion during *arisan* and *pengajian*, to health information sessions during the *posyandu* meeting. Texting creates a self-empowerment process that helps these women develop a strategy to maintain their multiple roles and sense of self-reliance (Chib & Chen, 2011) while dealing with hardships at the same time. Using common language, these women access the information they need and negotiate it with *mantri*—their main health supporter—and with other diabetics. At the same time, texting allowed these women to maintain their sense of self-reliance and ability to tackle hardships.

The practice of texting among the rural village women in this study shows us that health behaviors are rendered meaningful within cultural contexts, being anchored in cultural values and beliefs (Dutta, 2008). This study provides an insight into how a mobile phone can be used to help poor rural villagers or marginalized community members participate in the knowledge production related to health and illness. Recognition of local practices and traditions allowed these women's voices to be heard by *mantri* whom later elaborates on the health issues in his monthly health meeting or with the help of women volunteers in *arisan* and *pengajian* sessions. Culture, in the context of low-cost mobile texting, "emerges as the strongest determinant of the context of life that shapes knowledge creation, sharing of meanings, and behavior changes" (Dutta & Basu, 2007, p. 561).

References

Aikins, A., Boynton, P., & Atanga, L. (2010). Developing effective chronic disease interventions in Africa: Insights from Ghana and Cameroon. *Globalization and Health, 6*(6). Retrieved from http://www.globalizationandhealth.com/content/6/1/6.

Airhihenbuwa, C. O., Ford, C. L., & Iwelunmor, J. I. (2014). Why culture matters in health interventions: Lessons from HIV/AIDS stigma and NCDs. *Health Education & Behavior, 41* (1), 78–84.

Anwar, F., Khomsan, A., Sukandar, D., Riyadi, H., & Mudjajanto, E. S. (2010). High participation in the Posyandu nutrition program improved children nutritional status. *Nutrition Research and Practice, 4*(3), 208–214. https://doi.org/10.4162/nrp.2010.4.3.208.

Badan Pusat Statistik Indonesia. (2010). *Survey sosial ekonomi nasional (national socio-economic survey)*. Retrieved from http://catalog.ihsn.org/index.php/catalog/2260. Accessed March 15, 2017.

Badan Pusat Statistik, Provinsi Jawa Tengah/Central Statistics Bureau of Central Java. (2014). *Garis Kemiskinan Menurut Kabupaten/Kota (rupiah). 1996–2015*. Retrieved from http:// jateng.bps.go.id/linkTableDinamis/view/id/46. Assessed January 15, 2017.

Basic Health Research (Riset Kesehatan Dasar/RISKEDAS). (2013). *Badan Penelitian dan Pengembangan Kesehatan Kementrian Kesehatan RI, Indonesia*. Retrieved from http://www. depkes.go.id/resources/download/general/HasilRiskesdas2013.pdf.

Banerjee, A., Rathod, H. K., Konda, M., & Bhawalkar, J. S. (2014). Comparison of some risk factors for diabetes across different social groups: A cross-sectional study. *Annals of Medical and Health Sciences Research, 4*(6), 915–921.

Brenner, S. (1998). *The domestication of desire: Women, wealth, and modernity in Java*. New Jersey: Princeton University Press.

Central Bureau of Statistics, Minnesota Population Center. (2010). *Indonesian population census*. University of Minnesota. Retrieved from http://ddghhsn01/index.php/microdata.worldbank.org . Accessed February 18, 2017.

Chib, A. (2010). The Aceh Besar midwives with mobile phones project: Design and evaluation perspectives using the information and communication technologies for healthcare development model. *Journal of Computer Mediated Communication, 15*(3), 500–525.

Chib, A., & Chen, V. H. (2011). Midwives with mobiles: A dialectical perspective on gender arising from technology introduction in rural Indonesia. *New Media and Society, 13*(3), 486–501.

Chigona, W., Nyemba-Mudenda, M., & Metfula, A. S. (2013). A review on mHealth research in developing countries. *The Journal of Community Informatics, 9*(2). Retrieved from http://ci-journal.net/index.php/ciej/article/view/941/1011.

Cui, M., Wu, X., Mao, J. Wang, X., & Nie, M. (2016). T2DM self-management via smartphone applications: A systematic review and meta-analysis. *PLOSone, 11*(11). doi:10.1371/journal.pone.0166718.

Dutta, M. J. (2008). *Communicating health: A culture-centered approach*. London: Polity Press.

Dutta, M. J. (2011). *Communicating social change: Culture, structure, agency*. New York: Routledge.

Dutta, M. J., & Basu, A. (2007). Health among men in rural Bengal: Exploring meanings through a culture-centered approach. *Qualitative Health Research, 17*, 38–48.

Ferzacca, S. (1996). *In this pocket of the universe: Healing the modern in a central Javanese city*. (Unpublished doctoral dissertation). University of Wisconsin, Madison, USA.

Ferzacca, S. (2001). *Healing the modern in a central Javanese city*. Durham, NC: Carolina Academic Press.

Food and Agriculture Organization of the United Nations. (2016). *Use of mobile phones by the rural poor: Gender perspectives from selected Asian countries*. Retrieved from http://www.fao. org/3/a-i5477e.pdf. Accessed December 3, 2017.

Freedom House. (2015). *Indonesia freedom on the net*. Retrieved from http://freedomhouse.org/ sites/default/files/resources/FOTN2015_Indonesia.pdf. Accessed February 10, 2017.

Geertz, H. (1961). *The Javanese family: A study of kinship and socialization*. Glencoe, New York: The Free Press.

Green, L. W., Richard, L., & Potvin, L. (1996). Ecological foundations of health promotion. *American Journal of Health Promotion, 10*(4), 270–81.

Harper, T., & Amrith, S. S. (Eds.). (2014). *Histories of health in Southeast Asia: Perspectives on the long twentieth century*. Bloomington, IN: Indiana University Press.

Hsu, W. C., Boyko, E. J., Fujimoto, W. Y., Kanaya, A., Karmally, W., Karter, A., et al. (2012). Pathophysiologic differences among Asians, Native Hawaiians, and other Pacific Islanders and treatment implications. *Diabetes Care, 35*, 1189–1198.

Immajati, Y. (1996). *The Javanese women petty-traders in Salatiga, Central Java, Indonesia: Double female marginalization?*. The Hague: Institute of Social Studies.

Jay, R. R. (1969). *Javanese villagers: Social relations in rural Modjokuto*. Cambridge, MA: MIT Press.

Kaplan, W. A. (2006). Can the ubiquitous power of mobile phones be used to improve health outcomes in developing countries? *Globalization and Health, 2*(9). Retrieved from BioMed Central, http://www.globalizationandhealth.com/content/2/1/9.

Kitsiou, S., Pare, G., Jaana, M., & Gerber, B. (2017). Effectiveness of mHealth interventions for patients with diabetes: An overview of systematic reviews. *PLosOne, 12*(3). doi:10.1371/journal.pone.0173160.

Klansja, P., & Pratt, W. (2012). Healthcare in the pocket: Mapping the space of mobile-phone health interventions. *Journal of Biomedical Informatics, 45,* 184–198.

Koentjaraningrat. (1967). A survey of social studies of rural Indonesia. In Koentjaraningrat (Ed.), *Villages in Indonesia* (pp. 1–29). Ithaca, NY: Cornell University Press.

Kratzke, C., Wilson, S., & Vilchis, H. (2013). Reaching rural women: Breast cancer prevention information seeking behaviors and interest in internet, cell phone, and text use. *Journal of Community Health, 38,* 54–61.

Krishna, S., & Boren, S. (2008). Diabetes self-management care via cell phone: A systematic review. *Journal of Diabetes Science and Technology, 2*(3), 509–517.

Kreps, G. L., & Neuhauser, L. (2010). New directions in eHealth communication: Opportunities and challenges. *Patient Education Counselling, 78*(3), 329–226.

Kusujiarti, S. (1997). Antara ideologi dan transkrip tersembunyi: Dinamika hubungan gender dalam masyarakat Jawa. In I. Abdullah (Ed.), *Sangkan paran gender.* Pustaka Pelajar: Yogyakarta.

LIRNEasia. (2011). *Teleuse at the Bottom of the Pyramid 4 (Teleuse@BOP4).* Retrieved from http://lirneasia.net/projects/2010-12-research-program/teleusebop4. Accessed December 9, 2017.

Manderson, L. (1983). Introduction. In L. Manderson (Ed.), *Women's work and women's roles: Economics and everyday life in Indonesia, Malaysia and Singapore* (Development Studies Monograph No. 32). Canberra: Australia National University Press.

McKee, G., Clarke, F., Kmetic, A., & Reading, J. (2009). Health practitioners' perspectives on the barriers to diagnosis and treatment of diabetes in Aboriginal People on Vancouver Island. *Pimatisiwin: A Journal of Aboriginal and Indigenous Community Health, 7*(1), 49–64.

Mulder, N. (1996). *Individual and society in Java: A cultural analysis.* Yogyakarta: Gadjah Mada University Press.

Ng, N., Stenlund, H., Bonita, R., Hakimi, M., Wall, S., & Weinehall, L. (2006). Preventable risk factors for non-communicable diseases in rural Indonesia: Prevalence study using WHO STEPS approach. *Bulletin of the World Health Organization, 84,* 305–313. Retrieved from http://www.who.int/bulletin/volumes/84/4/305.pdf.

Parry, O., Peel, E., Douglas, M., & Lawton, J. (2006). Issues of cause and control in patient accounts of type 2 diabetes. *Health Education Research: Theory & Practice, 21*(1), 97–107.

Patrick, K., Intille, S. S., & Zabinski, M. F. (2005). An ecological framework for cancer communication: Implications for research. *Journal of Medical Internet Research, 7*(3), e23.

Pitaloka, D. (2014). *The (passive) violence of harmony and balance: Lived experienced of Javanese women with type 2 diabetes.* (Unpublished Dissertation). University of Oklahoma, U.S.A.

Pitaloka, D., & Hsieh, E. (2015). Health as submission and social responsibilities: Embodied experiences of Javanese women with type II diabetes. *Qualitative Health Research, 25*(8), 1155–1165.

Pujilestari, C. U., Ng, N., Hakimi, M., & Eriksson, M. (2014). It is not possible for me to have diabetes—Community perceptions on diabetes and its risk factors in rural Purworejo district, Central Java. Indonesia. *Global Journal of Health Science, 6*(5), 204–218.

Sallis, J. F., & Owen, N. (2002). Ecological models of health behavior. In K. Glanz, F. M. Lewis, & B. K. Rimer (Eds.), *Health behavior and health education: Theory, research, and practice* (3rd ed., pp. 462–84). San Francisco: Jossey-Bass.

Sears, L. (1996). *Fantasizing the feminine in Indonesia.* Durham and London: Duke University Press.

Shah, V. N., & Garg, S. K. (2015). Managing diabetes in the digital age. *Clinical Diabetes and Endocrinology, 1*(16). doi:10.1186/s40842-015-0016-2.

Soegijoko, S. (2009). ICT Applications in e-Health: Improving community healthcare services towards achieving the mugs. In *Proceeding for the United Nations Conference, Roundtable on Governance and Application of ICT for Achieving the MDGs*. Thailand, December 9–10, 2009.

Sojoy. (2014). *Dokter Diabetes* (diabetes doctor). Retrieved from http://www.soyjoy.co.id/ soylution/diabetes-and-me/496/dokter-diabetes-aplikasi-pertama-di-indonesia-untuk-konsultasi-diabetes.

Sujarwoto, S., & Tampubolon, G. (2016). Spatial inequality and the internet divide in Indonesia 2010–2012. *Journal of Telecommunication Policy, 40*(7), 602–616.

Sullivan, N. (1983). Indonesian women in development: State theory and urban kampung practice. In L. Manderson (Ed.), *Women's work and women's roles: Economics and everyday life in Indonesia, Malaysia and Singapore* (Development Studies Monograph No. 32). Canberra: Australia National University Press.

Sullivan, N. (1994). *Masters and managers: A study of gender relations in urban Java*. New South Wales, Australia: Allen & Unwin Pty Ltd.

Tickamyer, A. R., & Kusujiarti, S. (2012). *Power, change, and gender relations in rural Java: A tale of two villages*. Athens: Ohio University Press.

Utz, S. W., Williams, I. C., Jones, R., Hinton, I., Alexander, G., Yan, G., et al. (2008). Culturally tailored intervention for rural African Americans with type 2 diabetes. *Diabetes Education, 34* (5), 854–65. https://doi.org/10.1177/0145721708323642.

We Are Social. (2016). *Digital in 2016*. Retrieved from http://wearesocial.com/uk/special-reports/ digital-in-2016. Accessed March 12, 2017.

Wolf, D. (1994). *Factory daughters: Gender, household dynamics, and rural industrialization in Java*. California: University of California Press.

World Health Organization (WHO). (2016). *Global Report on Diabetes*. Geneva, Switzerland. Retrieved from: http://apps.who.int/iris/bitstream/10665/204871/1/9789241565257_eng.pdf. Accessed February 20, 2017.

XL. (2013). Xanesha diabetic analytic console. Retrived from http://www.xl.co.id/corporate/id/ ruang-media/info-perusahaan/xl-luncurkan-xanesha-diabetic.

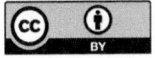

Chapter 5
Identifying Grassroots Opportunities and Barriers to mHealth Design for HIV/AIDS Using a Communicative Ecologies Framework

Jerry Watkins and Emma Baulch

Abstract The aim of this qualitative study was to test how social and cultural research methods can be used to anticipate opportunities and barriers to the use of consumer mobile devices by community health workers (CHWs) for HIV/AIDS prevention, testing and treatment. An exploratory study was conducted with CHWs (n = 19) at the regional capitals of Denpasar and Makassar in Indonesia in order to build to a clearer picture of how the participants have integrated personal mobile handsets into their daily professional and personal routine. A communicative ecologies framework was applied to the research design which included a range of qualitative methods including in-depth interviews, focus group discussions and communicative ecology mapping. Our main findings revealed that there was no bottom-up impetus for the introduction of a formal mHealth system to support client interactions. Existing client data collection systems were locked into paper-based systems to ensure compatibility with local government and/or funding body administrative systems; hence, mobile device-based data collection would require additional processes by the participants. Boundary issues were reported with regard to out of hours contact by clients. Some CHWs sent SMS medication reminders to clients but the strong preference indicated by all participating CHWs was to meet clients face-to-face in order to build and maintain trust through the in-person counselling process, rather than introduce mobile-mediated interaction.

Keywords Community health workers · HIV/AIDS · Communicative ecologies
Mobile phones · Indonesia

J. Watkins (✉)
School of Communication and Design, RMIT University Vietnam,
Ho Chi Minh City, Vietnam
e-mail: jerry.watkins@rmit.edu.vn

E. Baulch
Creative Industries Faculty, Queensland University of Technology, Brisbane, Australia

© Asian Development Bank 2018
E. Baulch et al. (eds.), *mHealth Innovation in Asia*, Mobile Communication in Asia:
Local Insights, Global Implications, https://doi.org/10.1007/978-94-024-1251-2_5

5.1   Introduction

This chapter reports on a bottom-up qualitative field study of everyday mobile device behaviours by HIV/AIDS community health workers (CHWs) in the regional capitals of Denpasar and Makassar in Indonesia. In contrast to the rural mHealth pilot described by Tariq and Durrani in Chap. 2, both sites of investigation feature comparatively good infrastructure in terms of mains power and network access, as well as ready availability of consumer mobile devices and affordable network tariffs. Hence, many of the barriers to scalability identified by Evans et al. in Chap. 3 (see Sect. 3.1) were not present at the sites of investigation in this study. Rather, all participants had personal mobile devices and most were at least moderate users of social networks. Therefore, the introduction of any consumer mHealth initiative at these sites which seeks to support health behaviour change across the lifespan will not only have to adapt to existing device and network availability and usage patterns but will also have to contend with the evolutions in devices and usage over the long-term.

As stated in the Introduction, a key aim of this book is to highlight how social and cultural research can play a more prominent role in understanding vernacular uses of mobile devices and their possible impact on mHealth programmes. In response to this aim, this chapter describes an exploratory study at two sites of investigation which used a communicative ecologies framework in order to build a clearer picture of existing mobile behaviours by CHWs working in the area of HIV/AIDS. This research was not conducted on behalf of or in association with any development agency or mHealth initiative; rather, our purpose was to test how social and cultural research methods can be used to anticipate opportunities and barriers to the use of consumer mobile devices to support lifelong healthy behaviours.

5.2   Problem Definition: Optimising Adherence to Therapy

Established HIV/AIDS communication strategies can focus on awareness-raising messaging campaigns in order to boost numbers of patients being tested and identified as disease-bearing. Whilst effective in attracting possible HIV+ clients to initial testing, this top-down approach to health communication is less focused upon retaining patients throughout the later phases of diagnosis and ongoing treatment to achieve suppression of viral load across the lifespan. Therefore, despite significant advances in HIV/AIDS treatment, a high percentage of people living with HIV/AIDS (PLWHA) do not maintain their programme of antiretroviral therapy (ART) and therefore do not achieve full viral load suppression. The UNAIDS Prevention Gap Report (2016) indicates that from an estimated 5.1 million people living with HIV/AIDS (PLWHA) in the Asia and Pacific region, an average of 34%

of diagnosed PLWHA continue antiretroviral treatment (ART) to full viral suppression.

This suboptimal percentage of retention of PLWHA in formal treatment continues to significantly degrade the long-term effectiveness of HIV/AIDS treatment in Indonesia and throughout the region. Provinces in Indonesia with high HIV/AIDS incidence include Bali, East Java, Central Java, West Java, Jakarta, West Papua and Papua (Jiamsakul et al., 2014). High-risk groups in Indonesia include men who have sex with men (MSM), female sex workers (FSW), clients of FSW, injecting drug users (IDUs) and so-called 'general women' (GW) (Republic of Indonesia Ministry of Health, 2012):

- *MSM* may be homosexual, bisexual or primarily heterosexual. It has been suggested that young MSM who are primarily heterosexual and cohabit with female partners may form a significant infection bridge (Walsh, 2011, p. 1861).
- *FSW*. Female sex workers occupy a high-risk category for HIV transmission. An interview-based study of commercial FSW in Bali reported very low levels of safe sex education and HIV transmission reduction skills, particularly in new FSWs who grew up in village environments (Januraga, Mooney-Somers, & Ward, 2014). The same study highlights the market pressure on FSWs to have unprotected sex with clients.
- *IDUs*. Unsafe injecting drug use is a major driver of both HIV and hepatitis C in the Asia region (Stone, 2015). The illegal nature of injecting drug use means that some IDUs may not disclose either drug use or HIV status when accessing health services. As a result, IDUs can 'have low HIV testing rates and, for those living with HIV, lower access to health services and lower viral suppression rates' compared to other PLWHA (Pierce et al., 2015).
- *GW*. 'General women' can refer to the heterosexual partners of MSM or male IDUs. This group may remain undiagnosed until symptoms develop or a child is lost due to HIV/AIDS; delayed detection in GW also impacts mother-to-child transmission as well as transmission to other partners (Rahmalia et al., 2015). A 2012 study forecasted that the GW group will become the second biggest category for new HIV infection in Indonesia after MSM (Republic of Indonesia Ministry of Health, 2012).

5.3 Grassroots Opportunities

In this context, the critical role of community health workers (CHWs) in supporting PLWHA to adhere to antiretroviral therapy across the lifespan) is clear. We uphold the discussion by Tariq and Durrani in Chap. 2 of this book regarding the critical function provided by community health workers (CHWs) within public health delivery (see also Perry, Zulliger, & Rogers, 2014). Our interest here is in exploring CHWs' everyday uses of mobile phones, and in considering such uses' promise for extending health services to marginalised groups.

A number of researchers have proffered assessments of mobile tools' potential to enhance the work of CHWs. According to Giachandani, for example:

...besides their increasingly ubiquitous use in patients' and caregivers' day-to-day lives, mobile and interactive real-time tools can enable community health workers to support their dual role as providers of health care to individuals and communities, as well as sentinels for emerging health hazards and needs (Gianchandani, 2011, p. 125).

To support this view, a thematic review of simple mobile-based communication tactics in low/middle-income countries found that one-way SMS or voice medication notifications and clinical appointment reminders were already a common application (Kallander et al., 2013). Such reminders can be sent directly to patients or to an intermediary such as a CHW, especially when a patient may not have mobile access or may not wish their identity to be known by formal health services —see, for example, DeRenzi et al. (2012). Two-way communication via mobile can include SMS requests for health advice or information on clinic locations (Déglise, Suggs, & Odermatt, 2012). Since the recovery regimes for both HIV/AIDS and injecting drug use (IDU) require the precise regulation of time to enable both daily medication and daily abstinence, these kinds of simple reminder services would be expected to provide a useful service to patients. Dutta-Bergman (2004) differentiates between active (requiring user motivation) and passive (minimal user effort required) channels of communication and even a simple mobile handset can offer access to passive support such as daily SMS reminders sent by a health facility or CHW.

With specific regard to HIV/AIDS retention, there is some evidence to indicate that adherence to ART can be improved through regular and early counselling that proceeds in tandem with mobile social networking. A monitoring study of 12 clinical sites from Hong Kong, Indonesia, Malaysia, Thailand and the Philippines identified multiple influences on suboptimal adherence within the first 2 years of ART including mode of HIV exposure, ART regimen, time on ART and frequency of adherence measurement (Jiamsakul et al., 2014). The authors propose that 'a greater emphasis on more frequent adherence counselling immediately following ART initiation and through the first six months may be valuable in promoting treatment and programme retention' (ibid.). In some contexts, CHWs can provide counselling services as either an accompaniment or an alternative to an outpatient facility. With regard to marginalised PLWHA, CHWs and community-based organisations can be particularly effective since social support from friends and family may be scarce due to the stigmatised nature of professional sex work or injecting drug use (Weaver et al., 2014). For instance, CHWs can give initial pre- or post-HIV test counselling and an introduction to formal health services as required; they can also provide longer term regular counselling to PLWHA in order to build and maintain adherence to ART over time (Jiamsakul et al., 2014). Alongside formal counselling services, in better-connected regions, mobile social networking can contribute to 'communities of support' understood as 'formally constituted, public structures such as support groups, self-help groups and mutual help groups' (Barnes, 2012). The importance of online communities of support to those with chronic illness with low access to resources is increasingly recognised (e.g. Davis & Calitz, 2016).

5.4 Grassroots Challenges

Despite the promise mobile technologies hold for extending outreach work for PLWHA, significant challenges remain. Previous studies demonstrate that mobile channels of health support are not necessarily adopted by PLWHA. From the patient's perspective, the receipt of regular SMS reminders—e.g. to encourage adherence to a daily ART regime or to support abstinence—may not be appropriate due to the perceived risk of 'discovery' by family, colleagues or others who may not know that the client is a PLWHA. For instance, a pilot test of mobile phone reminders (voice and text) to support adherence by 139 adult HIV patients at a Bangladesh clinic found that although 90% of participants reported the medication reminders as useful and did not perceive an intrusion of privacy, 87% reported a preference for a voice call over SMS (Sidney et al., 2012). These participants were largely urban-based and educated to at least a secondary level. A qualitative study of PLWHA participants conducted in Lima, Peru (n = 26) expressed positive perception of SMS reminders but with the significant proviso that the text replaced sensitive words such as HIV or antiretroviral with codewords or codephrases (Curioso et al., 2009). Furthermore, we should not assume that any SMS sent will actually be received: a 2014 interview-based US study (Gonzales, Ems, & Suri, 2014) argued that the multiple barriers presented by out-of-credit mobiles or by users who swap numbers regularly not only challenge simple communication strategies such as voice calls from health staff or automated SMS, they can also serve to further isolate the out-of-credit user from their wider online/mobile/social communities of support.

Neither should we assume that mobile-enabled systems will be embraced by all CHWs. A mixed-methods formative evaluation of an mHealth intervention at an HIV/AIDS clinic in Uganda found that some CHWs believed that mobile technology would threaten their jobs; others were uncomfortable with the confidentiality issues raised by having patient data on their mobile device, such as taking a patient's photo (Chang et al., 2013, p. 877). Also in Uganda, a study of a text message campaign that disseminated and measured HIV/AIDS knowledge in at-risk populations found that the design of the campaign 'failed to address several informational, economic, and sociocultural vulnerabilities' and that community-based research should be included as part of future campaign planning (Chib, Wilkin, & Hoefman, 2013, p. 30).

Even where support services such as outpatient visitation and/or CHW support are available, continuation of ART over the life course should not be expected. An interview-based study of PLWHA in Bali who also use drugs found suboptimal adherence behaviours in the participants despite comparatively good access to health services. Amongst other factors, participants cited ART side-effects, low viral load and apparent good health or 'knowing friends who had stopped treatment and were doing fine' as reasons for suspending or stopping ART (McNally, Mantara, Wulandari, & Lubis, 2013).

5.5 Aim, Sites of Investigation

The aim of this study was to test how social and cultural research methods can be used to anticipate opportunities and barriers to the use of consumer mobile devices by community health workers in the area of HIV/AIDS. Specifically, we investigated how CHWs have integrated mobile phones and social networking into their daily professional and personal routine—not as a result of a formal mHealth development initiative but rather through personal choice, organisational preference and/or in response to localised factors.

A qualitative study was conducted with participants from two community health NGOs in Indonesia. Participants were recruited from (a) the Yayasan Kesehatan Bali NGO in Denpasar, Bali and (b) the Ballata HIV/AIDS drop-in centre in Makassar, South Sulawesi. These two regional sites offered some useful comparisons for an exploratory study of this nature. First, both organisations were accessible to the research team and shared a similar core mission to mediate between local health departments and hard-to-reach, high-risk segments such as commercial sex workers and intravenous drug users living with HIV/AIDS. Second, the sites offered interesting contrasts: Denpasar (pop. $\approx$ 459 k at 2016[1]) is the capital city of Bali with a majority Hindu population. Denpasar is a rapidly developing business and tourism hub which attracts domestic and international tourists. Makassar (pop. $\approx$ 1.4 m at 2013[2]) is the capital city of the South Sulawesi region with a majority Muslim population. The city is a major commercial port.

Established in April 1999, Yayasan Kesehatan Bali (the Bali Health Foundation) is an NGO known more widely by the abbreviation Yakeba. Focusing on drug and alcohol addiction in and around Denpasar, Yakeba employs a team of field-based CHWs to

- Support drug users and people living with HIV/AIDS (PLWHA),
- Provide information about drug abuse and HIV/AIDS to clients and
- Facilitate client referrals to health services (Yayasan Kesehatan Bali, 2014).

Ballata is a drop-in centre in the city of Makassar, South Sulawesi where CHWs and outreach workers specialising in HIV/AIDS can share stories and information with colleagues. Ballata was established in 2012 as a provincial government initiative but today is maintained by a group of PLWHA and IDUs with various organisational affiliations.

---

[1]http://bali.bps.go.id/linkTableDinamis/view/id/20 accessed 20 July 2016.
[2]http://sulsel.bps.go.id/linkTabelStatis/view/id/115 accessed 20 July 2016.

5.6 Approach, Methods

Ten Yakeba community health workers or administrators were recruited (F4:M6) between 25 and 47 years old. Nine Ballata members were recruited (F3:M6) between 27 and 43 years old. Recruitment at both sites was facilitated a Bali-based NGO dealing with public information and journalism advocacy and with experience in HIV/IDU health communication. Regular use of mobile phones and social networks as part of the participants' work with PLWHA was a requirement for participation in the study. Two workshops were conducted with each group in the second half of 2013 at different locations in Denpasar and Makassar, respectively. All activities were conducted in Indonesian language. Research assistants took notes of interviews and group discussions. Where appropriate audio recordings were also made, parts of which were later transcribed. Where necessary some data were translated into English language for further analysis. Participants were offered a modest remuneration for their time contribution to the project.

The research design was constructed within the theoretical framework of the 'communicative ecology' which draws upon the fields of social anthropology, human–computer interaction and communication for development. The communicative ecology framework considers media usage at the site of investigation 'at both individual and community level as part of a complex media environment that is socially and culturally framed' (Hearn & Foth, 2007). Therefore, in order to understand any single aspect of a media technology intervention at a particular site, the communicative ecologies researcher needs to understand how the intervention fits into wider contexts. Furthermore, the research design had to be responsive to the range of issues arising from an investigation of this nature including client identity and data confidentiality and negative attitudes towards PLWHA from some elements of the wider community. In order to construct a research environment in which participants would be able to feel comfortable and to speak freely, three data collection methods were employed (informed partly by a study of HIV CHWs in Haiti, see Mukherjee & Eustache, 2007):

- Individual questionnaire on individual participants' use of their mobile phone, e.g. network, tariff, place most used (e.g. home, work and on the move) and principal activities performed (e.g. music, SMS, voice, gaming and SNS).
- Group survey on communication within the organisation (one interviewer per five participants). The survey consisted of four multiple choice questions on preferred formal versus informal sources of health management information (e.g. healthcare professional, social services, immediate family, friends, etc.) and four open questions on levels of trust in health information sources; self-perception of behaviour change due to health information sources; preference for health communication via phone, email or face-to-face; and the role of the mobile device in personal health management.

- Communicative ecology (CE) mapping (one interviewer per two participants). Informed by sociological work on communication and social order (Altheide, 1994), CE mapping is a conceptual rather than a cartographic method which connects a respondent's self-reported activity over a 'normal' 24-h to their communication behaviours during the same period, as part of an in-depth interview.

A second focus group was conducted 2 weeks later with the same group of participants. Participants were divided into two groups with one facilitator assigned to each group. Three main themes were explored during the workshops in order to generate further qualitative data on how each organisation has been impacted by mobile systems as well as the increasingly fuzzy border between personal and professional use of the mobile:

- *Impact of mobiles on work*: do CHWs find that having a mobile phone with them all day is generally a help—due to constant contact with colleagues, friends and family—or a hindrance—due to the stress of being always contactable?
- *Mobile versus in-person interaction*: to what extent can CHWs perform their work using mobile or other devices to communicate and share information? Do CHWs prefer dealing with challenging situations or clients in-person, by email or otherwise?
- *Personal connectivity*: to what extent do the mobile phone and/or social networks facilitate contact with friends and family? Maintaining personal connectivity can be an important support for those in counselling roles, especially since most of the participants from the Yakeba organisation were themselves in recovery and/or living with HIV/AIDS.

A manual thematic analysis was conducted on all data collected from the interviews, focus groups and communicative ecology maps in order to generate results. Four main thematic categories used for analysis are discussed below:

- Device and network usage,
- Impact of the mobile phone on work tasks,
- Preference for mobile phone versus in-person interaction and
- Personal connectivity with friends, family.

5.7 Results: Denpasar Site

5.7.1 Usage

Based on the individual questionnaire, seven out of ten of the Yakeba participants reported the mobile as their most important personal communication technology, and all participants considered the mobile to be of 'high importance' in their lives.

Analysis of the communicative ecology maps indicated different levels of device usage:

- Five participants reported that all their working hours and much of their waking hours were spent engaging with their mobile device for both professional and personal interaction. Two participants reported a feeling of confusion (*galau/bingung*) if they were unable to connect.
- Two participants reported the mobile device as their main daily communication technology interaction, which was restricted to a limited daily duration, i.e. each morning to confirm meetings and schedules.
- Two participants reported laptop usage as their main communication activity, one reported television.

The communicative ecology mapping exercise indicated that television was the second most-used medium, with all Yakeba participants reporting TV watching as a common night-time activity. Some reported consuming news and current affairs content whilst others had the television on as 'wallpaper'. Social media were widely used for work and/or personal networking including Facebook, Twitter, Foursquare and WhatsApp. Based on the responses from participants to the individual questionnaire on mobile device/social networking activities:

- Average spend on mobile credit was reported to be between IDR 100,000 and 350,000 per month.
- Eight participants used a BlackBerry (in some cases alongside a second Nokia handset).
- Eight participants used BBM (BlackBerry Messenger) as their main communication portal.
- Five participants checked their mobile immediately upon waking. Two participants checked their device in the early morning after domestic chores.

5.7.2   Impact of Mobiles on Work

The core philosophy of the Yakeba organisation is that people who have lived with drug or alcohol problems or who are HIV+ are best equipped to help clients with a similar condition or experience (Yayasan Kesehatan Bali, 2014). Therefore, a number of the Yakeba participants in this study were PLWHA and/or IDU, and a key feature of the NGO's culture was that co-workers should provide a mutual community of support to their colleagues. As a result, one of the most significant daily interactions reported by Yakeba participants was the daily in-person Narcotics Anonymous morning meeting at the main office. The daily message of support generated by this meeting was sent via SMS to staff unable to attend.

With respect to interaction between CHWs and clients, boundary issues were reported by some participants since some clients would contact Yakeba CHWs at antisocial hours, perhaps to ask for needles or for medication. Yakeba's Director had asked the CHW team to erect some boundaries in order to moderate such calls, e.g. that clients should warn CHWs when their ART supply was getting low, rather than waiting until their medication had run out to get in contact.

During the fieldwork for this project, the RIM BlackBerry was still the desired mobile device for much of the Indonesian market (Lee, 2014; Safitri, 2011) and partly as a consequence, the most popular network within the Yakeba organisation was the BlackBerry Messenger (BBM) app (although the BlackBerry is now being supplanted across Indonesia by the Android OS). The individual questionnaire flagged a gender-based and/or urban/regional digital divide within the participants: two female participants came from a regional area of Bali and had no BlackBerry, and hence no engagement with the various Yakeba activities facilitated by BBM— since BBM was only available on BlackBerry phones at this time.

5.7.3 Mobile Versus In-Person Interaction

A range of questions in the group survey responses on whether CHWs preferred to interact with clients via mobile phone (or other platforms) or via face-to-face meetings. An influential factor was the type of client with whom CHWs worked with. One CHW working with PLWHA stressed the importance of face-to-face meetings in order to accurately assess the health status of clients:

> I communicate most often face-to face, on a home visit. For example, some clients say on SMS that they are OK, but when you visit them, some cannot get up because of poor health. So we make sure of their condition by visiting them. (Translated response to group survey, 08 Sep 2013).

This was confirmed another CHW who stressed that phone communication with institutions, health departments or contractors was often inappropriate:

> To get to know a client's condition, I have to physically visit him... Furthermore, institutional meetings must be done face-to-face. (Translated response to group survey, 08 Sep 2013).

Those who did not work with PLWHA felt less need for face-to-face client interaction. One respondent pointed out that although BBM was a popular platform for internal communication, it did not extend to clients:

> To communicate with clients, I use the telephone and text messages the most. I rarely use BBM. Nowadays, clients rarely have or use BB. The intensity of my meeting with clients is also high. (Translated response to group survey, 08 Sep 2013).

The communicative ecology mapping exercise revealed that some core organisational interactions remained resolutely in-person. For example, the weekly team planning meeting remained a largely analogue affair: the agenda was circulated on paper, key weekly activities were written up on the whiteboard and staff members took notes on paper. Once the main aims and objectives for the week were established, individual staff members set up their appointments on BlackBerry or other available phones. In this way, the core business of Yakeba's CHWs and administrators remained similar to the pre-mobile system, i.e. in-person team briefings, paper-based agendae and notebooks and an emphasis on face-to-face interaction. New client data were captured on paper forms and then input onto spreadsheets or databases by a data entry operator employed by the NGO. Some client information such as contact details and a personal photo were maintained on the personal phones of CHWs; Yakeba's Director reported that the organisation had not received any complaints from clients about personal information storage despite the sensitivity of this information.

5.7.4 Personal Connectivity

Focus groups revealed that as well as communication with clients and colleagues, the mobile provided a social and emotional link to those Yakeba staff with family in other parts of Bali or Indonesia. When asked in the group survey about the impact of mobiles on their lives, some participants underlined the importance of their mobile phone and their main social network in connecting them to their family before discussing the use of the device for work. According to one team leader:

I use [BBM] to keep in contact with my family – many of my relatives live far away – but also to coordinate my team at work, to communicate with peers and with stakeholders at other agencies. (Translated response to group survey, 08 Sep 2013).

One CHW also spoke of the multiple ways in which she used BBM:

It's really useful for communicating with family, keeping in contact with clients and peers. I also use BBM to communicate with workers at the community health service. (Translated response to group survey, 08 Sep 2013).

During focus group discussion, two participants described their phone as their second wife/husband, suggesting a significant emotional dependence. Other social networks used for work and personal communication included Facebook, Twitter, WeChat and WhatsApp. Interaction with mailing lists was popular with one team leader:

...other than participating in the office group on BB, I also join in many other groups too... a high school group; my friends; my relatives; my extended family. For networking, I use WhatsApp, it has a networking group of Indonesian friends of drugs victims... I have joined many mailing lists. They can be accessed via my mobile phone. So, in one mailing list owned by PKNI [a national network of drug user organisations] many teenagers with HIV have joined in. A social-orientated NGO from Australia often posts comments there. (Translated response to group survey, 08 Sep 2013).

5.8   Results: Makassar Site

Nine participants from the Ballata organisation based in the city of Makassar were recruited for this study. Their occupations were as follows: field coordinator, project manager, PLWHA buddy (×3), community organiser and NGO activist (×3).

5.8.1   Usage

Ballata participants reported the expenditure of between 100 and 300 K rupiah a month on phone credit which was similar to the figures reported by the Yakeba participants. All participants reported that their employer did not pay for or sub-sidise their phone or online connection costs, although in some cases an employer did provide a laptop for work tasks. Two participants owned multiple handsets. Most of the participants used a low-cost access plan with cheap voice calls and in two cases, separate plans were used across different handsets to source the best price deals.

5.8.2   Impact of Mobiles on Work

One of the primary objectives of the Ballata organisation is to provide a support centre in Makassar where PLWHA can seek vital information from 'trusted friends' about the highly stigmatised HIV/AIDS condition. As a result, one important theme to emerge from the group survey was the question of which sources of health information were accessed and/or trusted by the Ballata participants. One group of participants pointed to friends, colleagues and family as the most trusted sources, whilst doctors and healthcare workers were mentioned by all participants as sour-ces. Due in part to a reportedly less-than-reliable mobile network availability, online desktops and laptops were used more frequently than mobiles for this kind of access. The reliability of online sources was an area of debate:

Facilitator:	[Scripted question and response options]. Where do you get information about health?
NGO activist:	I get it from the internet, friends, NGOs, community health centre and lastly from the doctor.
Comm organiser:	I get it from friends, internet, NGOs, community health centre and the doctor
NGO activist:	Friends, NGOs, internet, the doctor and the community health centre.
Outreach worker:	I get info from friends, then look on the internet, from NGOs, from the community health centre and the doctor.
Facilitator:	[Scripted question]. Which of these sources do you most trust?

Comm organiser:	Friends. Why friends? Because I think they are best able to keep a secret.
NGO activist:	Internet.
Facilitator:	Why?
NGO activist:	I don't have a reason, I just trust it.
Activist:	I trust colleagues, because they understand a lot of the information. Yep, friends and colleagues. I am with my friends every day. All the information that comes to me, I verify it on the internet, but that doesn't mean I get information from the internet, and swallow it whole. I just use the internet information to compare with what friends have said.
NGO activist:	I believe the internet. If you get information off people, you have to factor in human error.
Activist:	Do you really think there is no room for human error on the internet?! Who do you think puts this stuff on the internet?! Sounds like you really believe the internet, then!
NGO activist:	Yes, I believe the internet.

(Translated responses to group survey, 08 Dec 2013).

This exchange raises a number of important issues regarding health information literacy which are further explored in the *Discussion* (Sect. 4.8).

5.8.3 Mobile Versus In-Person Interaction

Both the focus group discussions and communicative ecology mapping indicated a common behaviour across participants:

- Voice calls were preferred for work conversations, e.g. with external organisations and stakeholders.
- SMS was used for personal communication but rarely for work.
- No social network or platform was used for inter-organisation communication.
- Face-to-face meetings with clients were preferred; in some cases, these meets were supported by voice calls to remind clients to take medication.

One Ballata CHW working with IDU clients suggested that face-to-face meetings were essential, since some IDUs did not trust the motivations of CHWs:

Developing a relationship of trust with IDUs takes a lot of time, because most of them assume that outreach workers are keen to move them into rehab, and many of them don't want to go to rehab. Many of them are scared of outreach workers for that reason. So cultivating a good relationship with them is a long process. (Translated interview comment by male community health worker, 08 Dec 2013).

For example, the Ballata project manager used email to coordinate frequent meetings with health department officials, whereas one of the NGO activists who conducted paralegal work frequently browsed via mobile in order to keep up-to-date with developments in criminal law related to drug use. No comparable use of a shared social network—comparable to Yakeba's used of BBM—was evident amongst the Ballata members, who worked for different organisations and had varying uses of mobile phones and Internet. Facebook was used by some participants for work contacts living in different regions including national bodies such as the National Drug Users' Union. The less-than-reliable network reported by the Makassar-based participants may be responsible in part for the lower use of mobile social networks when compared to the Denpasar-based Yakeba participants.

5.8.4 Personal Connectivity

Responses to the group survey revealed some complexity in personal device management. The BlackBerry remained a preferred device for some participants, in some cases operating alongside other brands such as Nokia and Samsung. One of the NGO activists reported a particularly complex device strategy in which the more familiar strategy of separating family and work contacts was approached rather differently:

Facilitator: [Scripted question]. What apps do you have on your phone?
NGO activist: WhatsApp, Line, WeChat. Initially I had a Fleksi phone [i.e.
                      CDMA handset]. Then I bought a BlackBerry and Android. Now I
                      use all three. Fleksi for my mum and my boss, because I am close
                      to them and often call them. The BlackBerry for friends who have a
                      BlackBerry. For my girlfriend and for work friends, I use the
                      BlackBerry.
Facilitator: Of those three devices, which is most important to you?
NGO activist: The Android. It has lots of apps.

(Translated response to group survey, 08 Dec 2013).

The PLWHA buddy also reported a multi-device strategy with a preference for social networking over voice and SMS:

PLWHA buddy: I use two phones, a Nokia and a BlackBerry. The BlackBerry is
                       for friends and groups and I have eight BBM groups. I also use
                       the BlackBerry for browsing, Twitter and WeChat.
Facilitator: Which do you use most?
PLWHA buddy: BBM. The Nokia is for voice calls and SMS.

(Translated response to group survey, 08 Dec 2013).

Another NGO activist reported a less 'complicated' device strategy which forewent mobile networking in preference for laptop access:

NGO activist:	I only have one phone. I'm the kind of person who doesn't want to be complicated. I don't want to use a BlackBerry and I only have a BlackBerry by coincidence. I used to have a Nokia but if they get wet, Nokias are hopeless. BlackBerrys are good, strong. I have had a Samsung for two years
Facilitator:	Can it access the internet?
NGO activist:	It can.
Facilitator:	What have you installed on it?
NGO activist:	Facebook and Twitter. But I don't use them. I access Facebook from my laptop. I just get notifications on my phone, so I can control my phone use.

(Translated response to group survey, 08 Dec 2013).

As indicated by the response from the NGO activist, the use of multiple devices by these CHWs cannot be understood using a simplistic segmentation such as the use of separate devices or social networks for family versus work. Furthermore, a multiple device environment also challenges the implementation of mHealth systems for CHW use. In principle, we could use a mobile web browser to facilitate compatibility across multiple mobile phones, but this could cause problems when the mobile cannot connect in low-/no-network reception areas which can be expected in the field. In contrast, the use of front-end apps might make offline work easier, but it may also require the implementation and maintenance of apps across multiple platforms. Assuming that some PLWHA clients also maintain multiple phones, the challenges multiply for even a simple system such as automated SMS medication reminders—how can CHWs and health authorities be sure that reminders are being sent to the correct device, that the device is in credit and is being monitored by the user?

5.9 Conclusion

Thematic analysis of the qualitative data collected from participants at both sites confirmed the ability of CHWs in both the Yakeba and Ballata organisations to mediate between health departments and hard-to-reach, high-risk segments such as commercial sex workers and intravenous drug users living with HIV/AIDS. Furthermore, the analysis demonstrated that the mobile phone was an important tool for CHWs at both organisations in terms of inter-organisation communication, supplementing or supplanting face-to-face interaction with clients, and maintaining important personal connections with friends and family. It has been suggested more generally that the possible application of mobile phones, networks and apps to community-level mHealth work 'has intuitive appeal' (Braun, Catalani, Wimbush,

& Israelski, 2013). However, this appeal must be weighed against some of the barriers to informal mHealth adoption by CHWs revealed at the two sites of investigation, to which other comparable organisations may be susceptible. Building upon the thematic analysis, the barriers discussed in this section are as follows:

- Health infrastructure,
- FSW client mobility and
- Information literacy.

5.9.1 Health Infrastructure

A number of policy reports have highlighted the need for the integration of mHealth solutions within a holistic healthcare delivery strategy (e.g. Lemaire, 2011). With regard to CHWs, it has been suggested that:

> End-to-end patient care systems and point-of-care support for health workers are needed whereby mHealth applications are interoperable and integrated with provider systems linking the most remote community health worker with the most appropriate sources of information when and where it is needed (Mechael et al., 2010, p. 5).

As a result, the effectiveness of the CHW is necessarily curtailed when the availability of a wider system of end-to-end care and point-of-care support is lacking, and there is only a limited amount that mHealth systems can achieve in such an environment. This barrier was illustrated well by the two contrasting sites of investigation selected for this study. The city of Denpasar is distinctive in that it hosts one of Indonesia's few drop-in HIV clinics for female sex workers, a very high-risk group. This clinic was also one of the few sites in the country where free access to ART medication for PLWHA was guaranteed. Access to medication and specialised clinics are two very important factors to longer term adherence to ART and from our analysis of data collected from the Ballata participants, it was inferred that access to ART medication was more limited for PLWHA in Makassar—which in turn limited the effectiveness of Ballata CHWs in keeping their clients on medication when compared to their Denpasar-based peers. In principle, ART medication has been free of charge for all Indonesians since 2006 (Jakarta Post, 2014). In practice, PLWHA have sometimes had to pay for ART due to insufficient supply of medication—and possibly some issues of graft in healthcare delivery (Buehler, 2008). Note that since the introduction of a new national healthcare scheme in 2013, there is evidence that the supply problems are being addressed: a 2015 estimate indicates 253 hospitals across 33 provinces where PLWHA can access free ART medication (Yayasan Spiritia, 2015).

5.9.2 FSW Client Mobility

CHWs are generally understood to be a member of the community in which they work (Kane et al., 2016) and by inference, it is understood that the CHW usually supports a geographically bounded population. Therefore, the *modus operandi* of all local health service providers—including CHWs—is challenged by a large transitory population which does not remain in one geographic location long enough to be able to connect with local health services. Although not specifically questioned on this point, the mobility of clients of HIV-infected female sex workers (FSWs) was raised by some Yakeba participants as a critical barrier to health service provision for HIV/AIDS. At the time of fieldwork, the Yakeba NGO had approximately 300 HIV and 90 IDU clients registered. However, the organisation's client numbers fluctuated monthly often due to infrastructure projects which can attract construction workers from other parts of Indonesia, in turn boosting demand for FSWs. For example, the Nusa Dua toll road project and the new Denpasar airport terminal were estimated by Yakeba to have brought 13,000 construction workers from Java into Bali between January and October 2013 as part of infrastructure spending catalysed by Bali's hosting of the 2013 Asia Pacific Economic Cooperation (APEC) Summit. It is extremely challenging for any regional NGO or health department to interact long-term with these highly transitory groups who may contract and spread the HIV virus to FSWs at their temporary work site and to wives and/or partners when they return to their home province. One can argue that the application of informal mHealth support could play a valuable role within this scenario via automated medication notifications or keep a transitory worker in touch with his/her own communities of support via social network. However, this would require the worker to be connected with mHealth providers in their home province, which may not be available in rural and regional areas. Based on group survey data from the Yakeba participants, other factors impacting client mobility include:

- Phased closure of recognised prostitution areas in Surabaya which increased the numbers of sex workers to Bali.
- Regular weekend movement of elite sex workers from Bandung and Jakarta to Bali in order to service clients.
- Increased MSM (men who have sex with men) activity during holidays.

5.9.3 Information Literacy

A primary function of the CHWs at both the Yakeba and Ballata organisations was to offer support and reliable health information to PLWHA from marginalised groups who might not have access to authoritative health sources either physical or online. For example, a qualitative study of newcomer FSWs working in Bali found a lack of knowledge and self-efficacy about HIV prevention due to low levels of sexual education, as well as limited opportunities to interact with positive social networks around HIV prevention (Januraga et al., 2014). Such lack of health information literacy is certainly not unique to HIV/AIDS—for example, see work on the potential of mobile dissemination of information on sexual reproductive health in Indonesia (Gerdts, Hudaya, & Belusa, 2014). The provision of reliable health information as part of wider education and awareness was identified as a key objective for a range of mHealth initiatives in developing countries (Chigona, Nyemba, & Metfula, 2012). However, the multiple issues that can arise when untrained users access unreliable online health sources are well known and despite the potential harm that inaccurate or misunderstood online health information can play in patient safety, many formal online health-related information accreditation schemes remain underused (Wong, Yan, Margel, & Fleshner, 2013). The pros and cons of online health information within the context of community health work were evident in the discussion between Ballata members (reported in the *Results* section). Although multiple sources of health information were accessed by most—e.g. Internet, friends, NGOs, community health centre and doctor—the participants differed on what they considered their most trusted source. One reported friends, one reported friends and colleagues, and one reported an unwavering belief in the Internet despite criticism from a colleague.

Information literacy issues were apparent at the Yakeba organisation in terms of client data collection and processing. As stated, new client data were captured on a range of paper-based forms since different funders of the NGO had different information reporting requirements. For instance, data required by the health department were manually input into a spreadsheet and then uploaded to a department website by a data entry operator employed specifically for this purpose by Yakeba. Although the Yakeba leadership was aware that this process could be substantially accelerated via off-the-shelf or customised mobile apps, their funding bodies preferred paper-based systems, and the NGO itself did not have sufficient funding or expertise to establish mobile data solutions. Furthermore, protocols for securing extremely confidential client data remained fledgling. When considering how even simple mHealth systems could support PLWHA to adhere to daily ART programmes, it is evident that systematised and confidential data protocols are required to generate and follow-up automated medication notifications or meeting reminders. Neither organisation studied was close to this level of information literacy. Two Yakeba coordinators stated that they saw no reason to move away from paper-based client data collection.

5.10   Conclusion

The aim of this qualitative study was to test how social and cultural research methods can be used to anticipate opportunities and barriers to the use of consumer mobile devices by CHWs working in the area HIV/AIDS. Through the application of the communicative ecologies framework and qualitative methods, we found no bottom-up impetus from either NGO for the introduction of a formal mHealth system to support client interactions. Although mobile phones were used extensively at both sites of investigation to support work-related functions, the clear preference for CHWs at both the Yakeba and Ballata NGOs was to meet PLWHA clients face-to-face in order to build trust and conduct an unobtrusive visual health check. There was limited use of basic SMS medication reminders by some CHWs but no organisation-wide automated systems to support ongoing adherence to antiretroviral therapy were in place. Client data collection was conducted using paper-based systems to ensure compatibility with local government and/or funding body administrative systems. Some team leaders at the Yakeba organisation saw little reason to replace the paper-based process with a more automated system which would require substantial reformulation of and retraining in data protocols not just by the NGO itself but also by local health departments and funding bodies. As community health services may often operate on a minimal budget, it was unlikely that any such reformulation and retraining would be available over the medium-term. Furthermore, the priority placed on face-to-face client meetings by CHWs at both the Yakeba and Ballata organisations would continue to physically limit the number of clients that each CHW could handle as part of their daily caseload, thereby limiting the possible efficiency gains via mHealth automation that a policymaker or funding body might seek when considering how to increase the financial sustainability of ART adherence and retention programmes.

One of the objectives of this book is to recognise that mHealth initiatives cannot be executed as technical programmes in a vacuum, ignoring the complex social and cultural contexts in which are implemented. Our study supports this view to some extent: by using a communicative ecologies framework to guide this study, we found that CHWs at both sites of investigation saw no significant opportunities for an mHealth intervention to improve their existing work processes or to more closely support client interaction. This is not to say that no such scope exists: rather, the significant organisational process changes that would be required by NGOs as well as local, regional and national health departments in order to introduce and maintain consistent mobile-friendly data collection, and security protocols would require resources that are not available at this time.

5.10.1 Limitations

This qualitative study was based upon two site-specific localised contexts which necessarily prevent any generalisation of the findings to a regional or national platform. Rather, this study should be considered alongside larger-scale quantitative reports such as the eHealth surveys conducted by the WHO Global Observatory for eHealth (WHO, 2016). However, our findings do confirm that multiple soft organisational and cultural barriers to adoption can be expected by any media technology-oriented project (Chang et al., 2013) and as a consequence, the adoption of formal or informal mHealth tools, methods or systems by CHWs and/or smaller scale NGOs should not be assumed by policymakers or system designers.

Acknowledgements We thank both the Yakeba and Ballata organisations for their full and open participation in this study. This research was funded by the Australian Research Council Discovery Project scheme *Mobile Indonesians*, DP130102990. Initial findings were presented both to the International Communication Association regional conference, Brisbane 01–03 October 2014 and the *Workshop on Mobiles and Social Media in Southeast Asia and the Pacific*, University of Sydney, 12–13 November 2015. We thank the reviewers who have provided feedback to earlier versions of this chapter.

References

Altheide, D. L. (1994). An Ecology of Communication. *Sociological Quarterly, 35*(4), 665–683.

Barnes, J. (2012). *Communities of support*. Paper presented at the IST-Africa 2012 Conference Proceedings. www.IST-Africa.org/Conference2012.

Braun, R., Catalani, C., Wimbush, J., & Israelski, D. (2013). Community health workers and mobile technology: A systematic review of the literature. *PLoS ONE, 8*(6), e65772.

Buehler, M. (2008). No positive news. *Inside Indonesia, 94*.

Chang, L. W., Njie-Carr, V., Kalenge, S., Kelly, J. F., Bollinger, R. C., & Alamo-Talisuna, S. (2013). Perceptions and acceptability of mHealth interventions for improving patient care at a community-based HIV/AIDS clinic in Uganda: a mixed methods study. *AIDS Care: Psychological and Socio-medical Aspects of AIDS/HIV, 25*(7), 874–880.

Chib, A., Wilkin, H., & Hoefman, B. (2013). Vulnerabilities in mHealth implementation: A Ugandan HIV/AIDS SMS campaign. *Global Health Promotion, 20*(1), 26–32.

Chigona, W., Nyemba, M., & Metfula, A. (2012). A review on mHealth research in developing countries. *Journal of Community Informatics, 9*(2).

Curioso, W. H., Quistberg, D. A., Cabello, R., Gozzer, E., Garcia, P. J., Holmes, K. K. et al. (2009). *"It's time for your life"*: How should we remind patients to take medicines using short text messages? Paper presented at the AMIA 2009 Symposium Proceedings.

Davis, D. Z., & Calitz, W. (2016). Finding healthcare support in online communities: An exploration of the evolution and efficacy of virtual support groups. In Y. Sivan (Ed.), *Handbook on 3D3C platforms: Applications and tools for three dimensional systems for community, creation and commerce* (pp. 475–486). Cham: Springer International Publishing.

Déglise, C., Suggs, L. S., & Odermatt, P. (2012). Short Message Service (SMS) applications for disease prevention in developing countries. *Journal of Medical Internet Research, 14*(1), e3.

DeRenzi, B., Findlater, L., Payne, J., Birnbaum, B., Mangilima, J., Parikh, T., … Lesh, N. (2012). *Improving community health worker performance through automated SMS*. Paper presented at the Proceedings of the Fifth International Conference on Information and Communication Technologies and Development, Atlanta, Georgia, USA.

Dutta-Bergman, M. J. (2004). Developing a profile of consumer intention to seek out additional health information beyond the doctor: Demographic, communicative, and psychographic factors. *Health Communication, 17*, 1–16.

Gerdts, C., Hudaya, I., & Belusa, E. (2014). *MHealth and safe-abortion: Improving information about and access to safe misoprostol abortions in Indonesia*. Paper presented at the 142nd American Public Health Association (APHA) Annual Meeting and Exposition 2014, New Orleans, USA. https://apha.confex.com/apha/142am/webprogram/Paper297938.html.

Gianchandani, E. P. (2011). Toward smarter health and well-being: an implicit role for networking and information technology. *Journal of Information Technology, 26*, 120–128.

Gonzales, A. L., Ems, L., & Suri, V. R. (2014). Cell phone disconnection disrupts access to healthcare and health resources: A technology maintenance perspective. *New Media & Society*, 1–17.

Hearn, G. N., & Foth, M. (2007). Communicative ecologies. *Electronic Journal of Communication, 17,* 1–2.

Jakarta Post. (2014, August 19). Domestically manufactured ARV medication warmly welcomed. Retrieved from http://www.thejakartapost.com/news/2014/08/19/domestically-manufactured-arv-medication-warmly-welcomed.html.

Januraga, P. P., Mooney-Somers, J., & Ward, P. R. (2014). Newcomers in a hazardous environment: A qualitative inquiry into sex worker vulnerability to HIV in Bali, Indonesia. *BMC Public Health, 14,* 832.

Jiamsakul, A., Kumarasamy, N., Ditangco, R., Li, P. C. K., Phanuphak, P., Sirisanthana, T., et al. (2014). Factors associated with suboptimal adherence to antiretroviral therapy in Asia. *Journal of the International AIDS Society, 17*(1), 18911.

Kallander, K., Tibenderana, J. K., Akpogheneta, O. J., Strachan, D. L., Hill, Z., ten Asbroek, A. H., et al. (2013). Mobile health (mHealth) approaches and lessons for increased performance and retention of community health workers in low- and middle-income countries: A review. *J Med Internet Res, 15*(1), e17.

Kane, S., Koka, M., Ormel, H., Otiso, L., Sidat, M., Namakhoma, I., et al. (2016). Limits and opportunities to community health worker empowerment: A multi-country comparative study. *Social Science and Medicine, 164,* 27–34.

Lee, T. (2014, October 02). BlackBerry losing popularity in Indonesia. *übergizmo.* Retrieved from http://www.ubergizmo.com/2014/02/blackberry-losing-popularity-in-indonesia/.

Lemaire, J. (2011). *Scaling up mobile health: Elements necessary for the successful scale up of mHealth in developing countries.* Retrieved from https://www.k4health.org/sites/default/files/ADA_mHealthWhitePaper.pdf.

McNally, S., Mantara, I. M. A., Wulandari, L. P. L., & Lubis, D. (2013). *Stopping ARV treatment in Bali, Indonesia.* Poster presented at the 11th International Congress on AIDS in Asia and the Pacific, Bangkok.

Mechael, P. N., Batavia, H., Kaonga, N., Searle, S., Kwan, A., Goldberger, A., ... Ossman, J. (2010). *Barriers and gaps affecting mHealth in low and middle income countries: Policy white paper.* Retrieved from http://www.comminit.com/ict-4-development/content/barriers-and-gaps-affecting-mhealth-low-and-middle-income-countries-policy-white-paper.

Mukherjee, J. S., & Eustache, F. E. (2007). Community health workers as a cornerstone for integrating HIV and primary healthcare. *AIDS Care, 19,* 73–82.

Perry, H. B., Zulliger, R., & Rogers, M. M. (2014). Community health workers in low-, middle-, and high-income countries: An overview of their history, recent evolution, and current effectiveness. *Annual Review of Public Health, 35,* 399–421.

Pierce, R. D., Hegle, J., Sabin, K., Agustian, E., Johnston, L. G., Mills, et al. (2015). Strategic information is everyone's business: Perspectives from an international stakeholder meeting to enhance strategic information data along the HIV cascade for people who inject drugs. *Harm Reduction Journal, 12*(41).

Rahmalia, A., Wisaksana, R., Meijerink, H., Indrati, A. R., Alisjahbana, B., Roeleveld, N., et al. (2015). Women with HIV in Indonesia: Are they bridging a concentrated epidemic to the wider community? *BMC Research Notes, 8,* 757.

Republic of Indonesia Ministry of Health. (2012). *Estimates & Projection of HIV/AIDS 2011–2016.* Retrieved from http://www.ino.searo.who.int/LinkFiles/HIV-AIDS_and_sexually_transmitted_infections_Estimates_and_Projection_HIV_AIDS_ENGLISH.pdf.

Safitri, D. (2011). Why is Indonesia so in love with the Blackberry? *BBC News.* Retrieved from http://news.bbc.co.uk/2/hi/programmes/direct/indonesia/9508138.stm.

Sidney, K., Antony, J., Rodrigues, R., Arumugam, K., Krishnamurthy, S., D'Souza, G., et al. (2012). Supporting patient adherence to antiretrovirals using mobile phone reminders: Patient responses from South India. *AIDS Care, 24*(5), 612–617.

Stone, K. A. (2015). Reviewing harm reduction for people who inject drugs in Asia: The necessity for growth. *Harm Reduction Journal, 12,* 32.

UNAIDS. (2016). *Prevention gap report.* Retrieved from http://www.unaids.org/sites/default/files/media_asset/2016-prevention-gap-report_en.pdf.

Walsh, C. S. (2011). *Mobile and online HIV/AIDS outreach and prevention on social networks, mobile phones and MP3 players for marginalised populations.* Paper presented at the Global Learn Asia Pacific.

Weaver, E. R. N., Pane, M., Wandra, T., Windiyaningsih, C., Herlina, & Samaan, G. (2014). Factors that influence adherence to antiretroviral treatment in an urban population, Jakarta, Indonesia *PLoS ONE, 9*(9).

WHO. (2016). *Atlas of eHealth country profiles 2015: The use of eHealth in support of universal health coverage.* Retrieved from http://www.who.int/goe/publications/atlas_2015/en/.

Wong, L.-M., Yan, H., Margel, D., & Fleshner, N. E. (2013). Urologists in cyberspace: A review of the quality of health information from American urologists' websites using three validated tools. *Canadian Urological Association Journal, 7*(100–6).

Yayasan Kesehatan Bali. (2014). *Yakeba—profile.* Retrieved from yakeba.org/?page_id = 111.

Yayasan Spiritia. (2015). *Daftar Rumah Sakit Rujukan AIDS di Indonesia.* Retrieved from http://spiritia.or.id/rsrujukan.php#SumateraUtara.

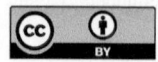

Chapter 6
mHealth, Health, and Mobility: A Culture-Centered Interrogation

Mohan J. Dutta, Satveer Kaur-Gill, Naomi Tan and Chervin Lam

Abstract In this chapter, we examine the interplays of the symbolic and the material in the constructions of mHealth. By attending to the key themes that play out in discourses of mHealth, we examine critically the ways in which power plays out in the structuring of mHealth solutions. The articulation of mHealth as instrumental to generating positive health outcomes in communities across Asia erases the contexts within which mobile technologies are constituted. mHealth interventions reproduce the logics of the state and the market, reproducing communities as homogeneous and monolithic sites of top-down interventions.

Keywords Mobility · Community · Neoliberalism · Mobile health

6.1 Introduction

Mobile platforms offer new opportunities for health communication scholarship. mHealth (or mobile health), which refers to the use of "emerging mobile communications and network technologies for healthcare," is an emerging innovation that capitalizes on the features and ubiquity of mobile phones across the globe to facilitate communication between patients and health institutions, to deliver health services, and to promote health preventive behaviors (Pattichis, Istepanian, & Laxminarayan, 2006, p. 3). The World Health Organization's global survey (WHO, 2011) reveals a range of uses of mobile technologies in health communications. Such technologies are being used to improve (1) communication from patient to health service providers (e.g., health hotlines or call centers); (2) communication from health service providers to patients (e.g., SMS reminders for appointments, compliance with treatments, or information to raise awareness); (3) health consultations over the mobile phone; (4) communication among health services in emergencies; (5) monitoring and surveillance of patient's health; and

M. J. Dutta (✉) · S. Kaur-Gill · N. Tan · C. Lam
Faculty of Arts and Social Sciences, National University of Singapore, Singapore, Singapore
e-mail: cnmmohan@nus.edu.sg

© Asian Development Bank 2018
E. Baulch et al. (eds.), *mHealth Innovation in Asia*, Mobile Communication in Asia:
Local Insights, Global Implications, https://doi.org/10.1007/978-94-024-1251-2_6

(6) the accessibility of databases of patient records (World Health Organization, 2011). mHealth applications in these areas of provider–patient communication, health services delivery, and health communication interventions promoting health behaviors have evolved globally. mHealth innovations from Asia have formed the cornerstone of narratives of Asian innovations in health care, circulated globally as markers of the power of mobile technologies in disseminating health.

On one hand, technologies such as mHealth are often discursively and materially constructed as the solution to health and social inequalities Asia faces today (Amrith & Amrith, 2016; Rama, Béteille, Li, Mitra, & Newman, 2014; Rhee, 2013), especially because of the large-scale penetration of mobile technologies in hard-to-access spaces in the region (World Bank, 2008; Kim, 2010). On the other hand, the concept of effectiveness of mHealth raises critical questions (Tomlinson, Rotheram-Borus, Swartz, & Tsai, 2013). However, missing from this literature is a theoretically informed framework for examining the flows of power, the structures of mHealth, and the concepts of communication that are embodied in mHealth solutions (Dutta, 2015). Beyond looking at the implementation of specific technology-based solutions offered under the framework of mHealth, it is worthwhile to examine the overarching power dynamics and interpretive frames that shape mHealth and constitute the textures of mobilities through mobile devices that deliver health and care. Particular to the Asian narrative of mHealth is the articulation of the power of mHealth in delivering health and care to under-reached spaces across Asia.

Both sides of the mHealth debate noted earlier posit technology as the elixir to structurally and spatially constituted problems of health and care (Dutta, 2015). These logics of health and care delivered through technology take-for-granted the larger structures that shape access to and utilization of health, and the terrains of power within which meanings of health are constituted and negotiated (Dutta, 2005). In this chapter, we draw upon the culture-centered approach (CCA) (Dutta, 2008, 2011, 2015) to interrogate the discourses of mHealth that frame health as a commodity to be delivered through privatized mobile technologies. As an alternative to this dominant discourse, we posit a culturally centered framework which aims not only to improve health outcomes in a narrow sense but also to foster communicative infrastructures for health justice. In CCA, the value of mobile phones for attaining and maintaining health and well-being lies not in their technical wizardry but in the ways they become embedded in existing patterns of mobility, vernacular health discourses, and locally constituted activist and advocacy movements seeking better health.

6.2   mHealth and Health Outcomes

Although mHealth in Asia has captured the interest and excitement of many scholars (Labrique, Vasudevan, Chang, & Mehl, 2013), the extent of mHealth's contribution to health outcomes in the region has been a source of contention. On one hand, proponents of mHealth attest to its effectiveness, often framing it as an omnipotent solution to problems of poor health in Asia (Istepanian, Laxminarayan, & Pattichis, 2006), and on the other hand, others are questioning the evidence for corollary health outcomes tied to mHealth (Tomlinson et al., 2013). This section explores the narratives of effects, examining closely the ways in which these narratives are deployed toward establishing the hegemony of transnational capital operating in the mHealth sector. Claims of effectiveness of mHealth in Asia serve as the basis of strategic mobile technology expansion, with limited attention to the health outcomes that can be attached to the grand claims of techno-modernity.

Given the great enthusiasm for mHealth and the significant investments poured into developing mHealth gadgetry and applications (Istepanian et al., 2006), it is unsurprising and inevitable that there is great hope in mHealth being useful. Tomlinson and colleagues (Tomlinson et al., 2013) opine that there is an enticing appeal to the concept of mHealth because it should, in theory, be effective, in removing the barrier of traveling for healthcare services. For the poor, this would entail a significant financial relief; they need not compromise a day's wage in order to travel, and those who cannot afford to travel need not. For those who are not poor, mHealth would bring about greater convenience, quicker access, and also quicker gratifications. At least, in theory, mHealth should deliver these benefits. There are findings that encourage this postulation; for example, in Indonesia, the *Midwives with Mobiles* project suggested that less skilled and remote community healthcare workers were able to deliver information to the centralized provincial hospital, via a JAVA-based mobile data delivery system (Chib, 2013). Bakshi et al. (2011) contend that mHealth is advantageous for developing countries because it requires low start-up costs and mobile phone services are affordable even to the poorest areas. For example, in India, there were more than 500 million mobile phone subscribers in 2010, and the rural subscriber base amounted to approximately 190 million (Shukla & Sharma, 2016). Shukla and Sharma also suggested some positive examples of mHealth; for example, the Health Information Helpline in India, which is a nonemergency helpline aimed at reducing the minor ailment load on the public health system, was a success and received over 70 million calls. As another example, Apollo, a private healthcare group, offered mHealth services to large numbers of Indians for as little as 2 cents per minute of phone call; consumers could call anytime and anywhere to get advice on medical or health queries from a panel of doctors (Shukla & Sharma, 2016). In Bangladesh, Khan and colleagues (Khan et al. 2015) found that mHealth was useful in addressing the country's shortage of trained health professionals; village doctors could call and get support and expert opinion from trained doctors. Thus, the use of mHealth is expansive and, in general, there is positive evaluation and expectation of its contributions to health outcomes.

Of note here is that the claims made in the above illustrations have more to do with health-related finance and time-saving outcomes than health outcomes per se. For example, there are very few pretest–posttest studies that show how mHealth directly improves the health of a community. In this sense, the methodological base for claiming effect is fairly weak. For instance, we lack a study that investigates the number of clinic visits within a community before and after implementation of mHealth services. Concrete cases of health outcomes derived from mHealth have been few and far between (Hall, Fottrell, Wilkinson, & Byass, 2014). Moreover, many of the proposed benefits of mHealth have been largely speculative in the literature (see Hall et al., 2014). For example, scholars may speculate about mHealth's potential in transforming health care (Steinhubl, Muse, & Topol, 2013), posit psychological mechanisms in using mHealth to combat obesity (Castelnuovo et al., 2014), recommend the potential use of mHealth apps for managing cannabis use (Norberg et al., 2015), or opine that mHealth has the potential to aid asthma self-management (Pinnock, Slack, Pagliari, Price, & Sheikh, 2007). However, such postulations remain largely unsubstantiated and there is yet to be concrete evidence justifying the use of mHealth, prompting scholars to pause for a "reality check" (PLOS Medicine Editors, 2013). In other words, the claims of large "effects" often remain unsubstantiated.

According to Tomlinson et al., (2013), there is little evidence regarding the likely uptake, efficacy and effectiveness of mHealth initiatives, many of which do not progress beyond pilot studies. Hall et al. (2014) concur with the dearth of evidence for health outcomes, suggesting that most 'evidence' related to mHealth is predicated on pilot studies and small-scale implementations and are sometimes merely anecdotal [see also Kahn, Yang, & Kahn (2010) and Gurman, Rubin, & Roess, 2012]. Chib (2013) posited that the majority of studies on mHealth in low income and low- and upper-middle-income countries have techno-optimistic views and have little theoretical support. The potential effectiveness of mHealth also appears to be contingent upon the environment it is employed in; mHealth may be more effective in a community that is technologically fluent, has strong organizational infrastructure, and has adequate resources to implement an mHealth initiative. In contrast, mHealth may not operate as effectively within a community that is not technologically proficient, is lacking in infrastructure, and has limited staff and finances to carry out an mHealth initiative. For example, an mHealth app that works with a community in New York City may not—and would most likely not—work as well in a different community, say, in rural India. As another example, Bullen (2013) suggested that implementation of mHealth in Cambodia would be challenging because of the country's system, culture, and dynamics; Bullen opined there were four hurdles: first, most Cambodians have multiple Subscriber Identity Module (SIM) cards, thus the frequent switching of SIM cards may compromise mHealth efforts. Second, most mobile phones used by Cambodians are not smartphones, and thus there are limited functionalities. Furthermore, most mobile phones do not support the national language, Khmer, and most Cambodians do not understand English. Third, many Cambodians do not own mobile phones but share phones instead. Fourth, as there is much unregulated commercial spam in Cambodia, phone users may mistake mHealth efforts as spam. Because the lived experiences, values, beliefs, and culture of "western" countries are markedly different from Asia, an mHealth app cannot be expected to replicate results from one to the other. Therefore, any mHealth effort must be tailored according to the culture in which it is employed.

Despite substantial scholarly critiques, the mHealth industry is rife with claims of miraculous effects, removed from the everyday lived experiences of communities with the health effects of mHealth. Moreover, the framing of Asia as a site for mHealth innovations paradoxically erases the cultural contexts that shape the meanings people make of the technology and the ways in which they interact with the technology in their lived experiences (Dutta-Bergman, 2005). In other words, the story of mHealth crafted in the dominant sites of knowledge production (international funders, academics in global organizations, mobile corporations, technology corporations, health corporations, civil society groups) on one hand reproduce the empirically removed claims about the transformative power of the technology, and on the other hand, obfuscate the cultural contexts within which the technology is constituted in the daily lives of community members. In the next section, we will interrogate the ways in which the concept of the community emerges in articulations of mHealth.

6.3 mHealth and Community

The mobile phone has been studied as a tool that has the potential to narrow the digital divide, specifically across communities that are typically disenfranchised and resource poor. Community therefore emerges as a conceptual category in the framing of mHealth. With the popularization of the mobile phone across the globe and more specifically in Asia, the mobile phone today is available and affordable to almost all strata and socioeconomic classes in many societies of Asia. This claim of the ubiquity of mobile phones in Asia forms the bedrock of the knowledge claims of mHealth. To illustrate, the mobile phone is used by a large proportion of the Indian population, including 16.6 million rural users that consists of new subscribers each month (Cumiskey & Hjorth, 2013). Similarly, in the Philippines, connectivity of mobile phones in sparse and topographically challenging regions are common, with prepaid mobile services more common among low-income users (Zapata, 2016). Zapata (2016) thus, opines that "the pervasiveness of the mobile phone even in remotest communities is noteworthy of attention" (p. 4).

The adoption of the mobile phone has led to the belief that mHealth interventions can be potentially transformative for communities where healthcare services may be relatively inaccessible (Cumiskey & Hjorth, 2013). Asia has seen a significant number of mHealth interventions for the purposes of enacting behavior modifications for better health outcomes (Gurman et al., 2012). mHealth has been recognized as a technological advancement that has the potential to reshape the ways in which health services can be consumed by different segments of populations and communities in Asia that are often demographically, socially, and culturally, heterogeneous. This means having to provide a range of healthcare services that meet a wide variety of needs across diverse spaces, including previously hard-to-reach communities (Fiordelli, Diviani & Schulz, 2013; Khatun, Heywood, Ray, Bhuiya, & Liaw, 2016).

Observing the growth of the mobile phone in various communities around the world, many medical and public health scholars see mHealth as potentially impactful in the delivery of healthcare services, especially in communities that face significant challenges accessing healthcare services for a myriad of reasons that will be discussed further in this chapter (e.g., Malvey & Slovensky, 2014; Olla & Shimskey, 2015; Post et al., 2013; White, Thomas, Ezeanochie & Bull, 2016). Malvey and Slovensky (2014) view mHealth as having an emancipatory potential in terms of the delivery of healthcare services for hard-to-reach communities around the globe, opining that current research has indicated that there has already been good consensus among patients and community health workers regarding the desire for provision of healthcare services through mHealth avenues (e.g., Chang et al., 2013; Nachega et al., 2016). Explaining the global interest by medical and public health scholars to implement mHealth applications in a bid to deliver healthcare services in areas with socioeconomic and geographical challenges in accessing good healthcare systems, infrastructures, and knowledge, scholars emphasize the emancipatory power of mHealth (Chang et al., 2013). A pervading discussion on mHealth in Asia relates to the viability and sustainability of mHealth interventions in communities that may often use texting or health applications to aid in patient care across a variety of health contexts, such as sharing educational resources with communities and the community's health workers often situated within nonurban centers (Atun, 2012; Chang et al., 2013; de Jongh, Gurol-Urganci, Vodopivec-Jamsek, Car, & Atun, 2012). These include rural and remote villages that may be geographically and topographically hard to access. Inherent then in the dominant notions of mHealth, are techno-deterministic notions of mHealth technologies as instruments for delivering health solutions devised by experts at knowledge centers (e.g., Manda & Sanner, 2014; Kay, Santos & Takene, 2011).

The role of community healthcare workers includes maintaining continued support in health decision making of these hard-to-reach communities. The scope of mHealth in Asia includes reaching out to remote communities on infectious diseases, chronic diseases, and maternal, and prenatal care. Community healthcare workers also support better provider–patient interaction for health decision-making among patients that may not typically have formal healthcare facilities (Chang et al., 2013; Atun, 2012). Community healthcare workers are an important stakeholder in mHealth success in Asia and are said to benefit significantly from mHealth services when working in isolated spaces. White et al. (2016) adopted a systematic review on healthcare workers' utilization of mHealth and found that workers were highly accepting of mHealth, and saw it as having important benefits for all stakeholders involved. Studies consistently indicate that mHealth has the potential to increase patient compliance if community health workers acquired and adopted mHealth technologies positively to better communicate with patients. However, sustainability issues of these technologies are still a challenge (White et al., 2016). Katz, Mesfin, and Barr (2012) found that mHealth was useful in the management of chronic disease among low-income patients. Upon investigating factors that contributed to the success of the technology in health outcomes, the study found that success or failure depended on the role of the community healthcare workers' involvement in mHealth as opposed to the design, interface, or specific qualities of the technology itself. Additionally, in resource-constrained Asian countries that do not have substantially trained healthcare providers, community healthcare workers adopt mHealth technologies for instruction and guidance from experts such as doctors and nurses when dealing with patients and their care. In many Asian countries that make up the global south, mHealth projects are gaining traction as mHealth technology is seen to empower workers situated in rural areas through increasing knowledge, skills, and supervision, while integrating these workers in the national healthcare system. They are also trained in assisting with patient referrals and follow-up treatments (Khokhar, 2009; Watterson, Walsh, & Madeka, 2015).

Both community health workers and patients recognize that mHealth can alter the quality of patient care positively, but studies in these areas have found significant challenges and barriers that impede the use of mobile technology in delivering health services. These include inconsistencies in the kinds of smartphones used by community healthcare workers that lead to poor imaging of the condition, which in turn, causes difficulties in assessing and diagnosing patients (Asgary et al., 2016; Free et al., 2013). Additionally, a systematic review of mHealth interventions on community healthcare workers found that most interventions were overwhelmingly focused on the context of the global North, with many of them having limited success outside of that space (Free et al., 2013). Missing from these studies are the cultural contexts, and more specifically, the cultural contexts of Asia. Bangladesh is a popular example, since—with more than 20 current initiatives—mHealth is valued as a potential supplement to an over-burdened healthcare infrastructure which faces a significant shortage of healthcare workers (Khatun et al., 2016). In such celebrations of mHealth among communities in Asia however, the very notion of communities and their local contexts remain mostly absent.

6.4 mHealth and Hard-to-Reach Communities

mHealth technology has been used to mobilize health messages that range from inducing knowledge to increasing participation in campaigns that involve screening, immunization, or counseling among hard-to-reach communities. Essential to these articulations of mHealth technologies is the positioning of communities at the margins as recipients of expert solutions, carried by mobile technologies. These top-down, expert-designed health messages are meant to induce positive behavioral modifications among communities that may typically not have knowledge or access to such facilities, without institutionalized message dissemination (Kay et al., 2011). Despite mHealth being implemented in a variety of communities battling different medical challenges, studies on effectiveness and health outcomes have not been promising, regardless of the desire by communities to adopt the intervention (Chib, 2013; Tomlinson et al., 2013). Moreover, the conceptualization of "hard-to-reach" communities frames these communities as inaccessible, constituted in the language of information deficit. Framing communities through the lens of inaccessibility perpetuates models of communication that are typically asymmetrical (Atkin & Wallack, 1990; Lupton, 1994), bulleting messages through tools of technology to modify individual behavioral change in these unworkable spaces. To add, the very theorizing of behavioral change as an individualistic act begins by already negating other key factors involved in the matrix of inequality and inaccessibility (Dutta-Bergman, 2005). Thus, experts removed from the communities and their experiences with mHealth, are in control of developing matrices and measuring change through individual behavioral indicators (Dutta, 2008, 2015).

Due to the nature of evaluation that focuses on behavioral change at the individual level, many studies investigating the use and efficacy of mHealth by communities have found a variety of challenges communities face when using different mHealth services. Despite high mobile penetration rates, low literacy levels affect how the mobile phone is used. Text messaging or using the mobile phone for the Internet may not always be functional for some populations, causing a lack of competency or misunderstandings in mHealth use (Agarwal, Perry, Long & Labrique, 2015; Chib, 2013; Khatun et al., 2016). Studies have also found that mHealth applications tended to be preoccupied with technical functions, as opposed to usability and content of the technology centered on the needs of the community using the technology (Schnall et al., 2016). The cultural threads of the community and their ways of knowing and understanding are secondary to the conceptualization of the application, which often leaves mHealth applications redundant or limited in use by communities. These cultural threads such as gender roles, collectivistic epistemologies of knowing, living, and understanding, and/or power denominations in communities are just a few ways to think about the heterogeneity that exists across communities, and their relevance in making sense of how mHealth comes to be shaped in communities. Studies looking at mHealth and culture, reflect these challenges. Khatun et al. (2016) discusses the inability to use mHealth services by some Bangladeshi women without seeking permission from their spouses. These challenges force researchers to think through questions tied to culture, in the enactment of privacy and security as valuable in the designing of mHealth applications (Bajwa, 2014). In other scenarios, certain communities were found to have preferences for mobile phone functions such as voice communication instead of text messaging (Thomsen et al., 2016).

In studying a remote village *Chakaria* in Bangladesh, researchers found that village doctors, who constituted the informal healthcare providers for village members, sought knowledge through call centers run by formal doctors. This system was extremely useful in this setting where there were significant shortages of formal healthcare providers. Village doctors, however, reported challenges such as inaccessibility and unfamiliarity with the technology and with the formal doctors that were working with them through the call centers (Khan et al. 2015). Among vulnerable communities, uncertainty of mHealth applications may further inhibit use. Nachega et al. (2016) found HIV-infected pregnant mothers feared unintended or accidental disclosure, and therefore had specific expectations, such as alerts and reminders they wanted to be sent within specific hours of the day. The specificity of timings regarding these alerts had to do with managing their privacy, so as to prevent their status as HIV-infected pregnant mothers from being disclosed. mHealth in Asia is also seen as a potential technology to overcome mental health stigmas, where mental health and suicide are viewed negatively. Note in these studies the absence of culture on the one hand, and the instrumental logics of conceptualizing culture on the other hand. The cultural spaces of community life and the meanings of health in these cultural spaces remain erased from the configurations of mHealth, turned into targets for top-down, expert-driven interventions.

Top-down understandings of how technology is used fail to account for the nuances in mediation of technology use and its manifestations in communities that have alternative ways of understanding and conceptualizing technology (Zapata, 2016; Chib, 2013). Jennings et al. (2016) therefore conclude that for mHealth interventions to be successful, communities must be engaged right from the onset of the intervention design, to fully understand the contextual and community complexities in health barriers, before moving into the distribution of mHealth services. As communities are largely shaped by these structural and cultural variances, mHealth application must assess and locate these differences in order to successfully develop an intervention that is meaningful and viable for hard-to-reach communities. Hall et al. (2014), after conducting a systematic review of mHealth among middle- and low-income communities, posit that mHealth continues to show positive signs for future interventions that are feasible for resource-poor communities. However, these claims of mHealth and their effectiveness in impacting community health outcomes ought to be situated within broader discussions of technology, state, and the market. Contemporary health discourses individualize health responsibilities and unburden states from addressing health disparities, depicting the overarching neoliberal ideology of organizing health (Dutta, 2015). By adopting techno-optimist solutions, such as mHealth, as solutions to inequalities, states can justify allocation of resources to the margins as inefficient, leaving the broader structures of inequality intact (Dutta, 2015).

6.5 mHealth, State, and Market

International organizations such as the United Nations, World Health Organization, and World Bank have expressed support for the implementation of mHealth initiatives to meet the Millennium Development Goals and are promoting such programs to member countries (WHO, 2011). In these neoliberal narratives of global health, mHealth's intrinsic relationship with mobile phone technologies represents immense opportunities for bridging health disparities, obfuscating conversations on the fundamental barriers in terms of access for disenfranchised or hard-to-reach communities (Dutta, 2015). The mHealth literature thus far has tended to highlight only the potential of mobile phones in improving health outcomes of patients, but has yet to address broader structural issues, limitations, and pitfalls to do with the uncritical adoption of this new communication technology (Kaplan, 2006; Levin, 2012; Malvey & Slovensky, 2014; McBride & Rimer, 1999). The framing of the state as a facilitator of market-based solutions of mobile health technologies takes-for-granted the very inequities in health outcomes that are produced by the large-scale penetration of these technologies into communities at the margins (Dutta, 2015).

In the dominant framework of mHealth, the role of the state is seen as crucial in building up the appropriate health applications or systems and communication infrastructure in order to support the use of mHealth and to harness its potential. As of 2014, Asia was the region with the highest number of mHealth and eHealth program implementations, driven by government investments in the healthcare sector (Healthcare Asia, 2014). However, it is estimated that only 67% of rural inhabitants globally are covered by a mobile-broadband network, compared to 84% of the general population (ITU, 2016). In the Asia Pacific, only 42.6% of the population have a mobile-broadband subscription, and the percentage of online users who have access to high-speed broadband in the developing world is substantially lower compared to developed countries (ITU, 2016). These statistics need to be further tempered by issues such as language and illiteracy, mobile phone literacy, and gender gaps in mobile phone ownership and usage, which affect the adoption of mHealth in Asia (Mechael, 2009). Therefore, despite the high number of mHealth programs being implemented, there remain fundamental structural and knowledge barriers that have yet to be addressed (Kaplan, 2006). On one hand, the prevalence of mHealth programs in Asia could reflect the popularity (and by extension, effectiveness) of such initiatives; on the other hand, this could also be indicative of the piecemeal nature of mHealth implementation in Asia, which could be in part due to a lack of proper infrastructure. Moreover, the very development of such infrastructure by the state deploys the logics of health to create new opportunities for privatization through new markets comprising of the poor and the underserved. The technology-driven agenda of the state shifts attention away from the role of the state in addressing social determinants of health upstream and healthcare structures and resources downstream.

The rise in popularity of mHealth has also resulted in a lucrative industry consisting of organizations, small to large, that build health applications and technology (Malvey & Slovensky, 2014; Schweitzer & Synowiec, 2012). It is estimated that the mHealth industry will grow to US$23 billion by 2017 (PricewaterhouseCoopers, 2012). While some initiatives are not-for-profit, most are profit oriented, such as the creation of technological products and applications which could be sold and used in developing countries. Large multinational companies such as Johnson & Johnson, Merck, and GlaxoSmithKline are also increasing funding for mHealth projects in various parts of the world (Qiang, Yamamichi, Hausman, & Altman, 2011). Droppert and Bennett (2015) described how corporate social responsibility (CSR) initiatives are often tied to broader business objectives of companies and are strategized as an investment for future growth in the region. For example, representatives from pharmaceutical companies reported that their motivations for CSR include building up a country, its population, and its economy to prime the region for future economic expansion, or as a way to do market research which informs their business decisions (Droppert & Bennett, 2015). Health thus is diverted by the state into a new market opportunity for transnational capital, bringing together mobile technologies with health commodities. The state is reworked as an enabler of private capital, ensuring profits for both the bio and mobile technology industries.

While some initiatives are small-scale, informal, community-based, or disease/treatment-specific, others are scalable and integrated with formal health systems or telecommunication companies. Many of the initiatives are supported and funded by international organizations and universities. For example, the mCARE program aims to decrease infant mortality in rural Bangladesh by providing expectant mothers with mobile phones. This initiative, which is funded by USAID, the Bill and Melinda Gates Foundation, and the US Department of Agriculture, allows mothers to inform their health workers once they go into labor so that necessary medical treatment can reach the mother and child in a timely manner (Johns Hopkins Bloomberg School of Public Health, 2012). The interplays of imperial aid agencies, foundations, and the development sectors constitute an overarching framework of health that is fundamentally grounded in the individualization of health. In another example, CycleTel Humsafar, is a free SMS service in India introduced by the Institute for Reproductive Health (IRH) at Georgetown University and USAID. This service helps women and their partners with family planning using the "Standard Days Method" or the rhythm method. It also includes a family advice component, which is available through Nokia Life, an application only available through Nokia mobile devices. Note here the interplay of the logics of private capital with the agendas of private foundations, global development agencies and the nation-state.

Similar to CycleTel, many mHealth applications are the result of public–private partnerships (Schweitzer & Synowiec, 2012; WHO, 2011). In particular, telecommunication companies appear to be leveraging the potential of mHealth to provide health services that are pitched as significantly less costly compared to a visit to the doctor. In rural India, the telecommunications company Ericsson has partnered with Apollo Hospitals Group's Apollo Telemedicine Networking Foundation in 2008 on an mHealth initiative that brought medical information and health advice to populations in remote villages and towns (Ericsson, 2008). This initiative was also intended as a way to promote the use of telemedicine through mobile phone applications to these hard-to-reach communities (Ericsson, 2008). In the Philippines, the leading telecommunications company and mobile operator, Smart Communications, is a key player in the local mHealth market. Smart Communications launched SHINE, Secured Health Information Network and Exchange, an integrated health information system that connects different stakeholders. The company also worked with the government to provide an SMS service that delivered health information to its users (Handford, 2012). Health as a commodity enables the networks of mobile profiteering, catalyzed through state-based initiatives and public–private partnerships. The onus of delivery of health is privatized, having been converted into a new market opportunity, while simultaneously pushing new markets for private capital in the mobile technology sector.

The examples presented here are a small slice of the mHealth technology that is available on the market today. mHealth applications are diverse in their functionalities; while some apps leverage on relatively simple features of the mobile phone (i.e., SMS and voice call functions), other companies are using cutting-edge technology to meet the health needs of users. For instance, Samsung's S Health app enables users to perform a whole range of activities, including monitoring one's heart rate, with the potential to connect to medical devices (Comstock, 2014). Such mHealth apps that monitor and store data raise important concerns regarding data security and privacy of patient's health information with the advent of mHealth technologies. Given that one of the common goals in the industry is the creation of an ecosystem that integrates mHealth with formal health systems in each country, the role of the state in establishing laws and policies protecting patients' right to data privacy is imperative (Malvey & Slovensky, 2014). This includes regulations on which data are collected, how they are stored and transferred, and who has access. According to a report by the mHealth Alliance (2013), a possible regulatory framework must include (1) informed consent and choice to opt-in; (2) data minimization to reduce the risk of loss of privacy; (3) patients' accessibility to personal data; (4) laws on data security; (5) limit transfer of data across jurisdictions; and (6) enforcement of laws and regulations. More importantly, critical conversations ought to attend to the role of the state in enabling the movement of capital and profits in health across Asia.

6.6   Conclusion

Articulations of mHealth in Asia are situated within the logics of health tied to frameworks of global capital flows. In the conceptualizations of mHealth in Asia, health emerges as a market-based commodity to be delivered through privatized mobile technologies. The movement of health from the centers of knowledge production to distant spaces in Asia through mobile technologies is constituted in the erasure of culture and community as sites of meaning making. Expert knowledge developed in networks of power is disseminated through mobile technologies into hard-to-reach communities. Mobile technologies enable the reach of capital into subaltern spaces of Asia, premised on the delivery of the miracles of health and wellbeing. The ideology of mHealth is empirically empty, removed from the evidence of health effects of mobile technologies. The lack of empirical evidence translates into large claims about the possibilities unleashed by mobile health in Asia. The power ascribed to technology and its ability to uplift the "burden of the soul" is disengaged from empirically grounded studies that enable cause-effect claims. Moreover, the articulation of mobile health in Asia rests on the framing of community as resources for health delivery, at the same time, treating the notion of community as a monolith. Community emerges in narratives of mHealth in Asia as a monolithic receptacle of mHealth interventions, enabled by community health workers, catalyzed to deploy the mobile technologies of health. Moreover, the positioning of mHealth as solutions to problems of health inaccess drives the active role played by the state in enabling the commoditization of health into new markets for mobile technology corporations. CSR and public–private partnerships deliver new opportunities for expansion of privatized mobile companies, wrapped up in the age-old seductive appeal of technology as an instrument of development.

How can we then move towards democratizing technologies such as mHealth that can engage with communities in resourceful ways? CCA theorization begins by first unpacking development discourses embedded in the distribution of technologies, uncovering the ways in which top-down effects of technology are sold as enabling better health while at the same time commoditizing health to push market opportunities. Moving forward, the CCA pushes researchers to situate mHealth amidst local expressions of the relationships between structure and culture, foregrounding community agency through collective organizing and advocacy to challenge the neoliberal structures of healthcare. Thus, a CCA scholar interrogating mHealth and its applications might begin by asking local communities, what are the ways in which they face health injustices? By doing so, the researcher first begins by recognizing the agentic capacities of a community to articulate their structural limitations in accessing and achieving better healthcare systems, and in organizing their own mHealth interventions (agency), designed to account for their community and health needs. Cultural and structural articulations are located within the sites of technological interventions, described by those that can best represent their health concerns. Zapata (2016) for example, studies mobile phone and indigeneity using the CCA as a framework. She describes the various dialectics of mobile phone use, suggesting its role in complexifying indigeneity in the community, yet being extremely useful in coordinating community health issues. By making sense of how technology is mediated in cultural spaces in collaborative and dialogic ways, we move away from interventionist approaches of technology use, and instead, toward communizing spaces where communities can contest the meanings of technology and its uses, centering their own articulations of their relationship with technology. In recognizing the polemical in disenfranchised spaces, CCA theorizes the inter dependent ways the meanings of technology use come to be located, reworking technology in community networks as sites for solidarity building and resisting neoliberal capital.

References

Agarwal, S., Perry, H. B., Long, L., & Labrique, A. B. (2015). Evidence on feasibility and effective use of mHealth strategies by frontline health workers in developing countries: Systematic review. *Tropical Medicine and International Health, 20,* 1003–1014. https://doi. org/10.1111/tmi.12525.

Amrith, M., & Amrith, S. (2016). Migration, health and inequality in Asia. *Development and Change, 47*(4), 840–860.

Asgary, R., Adongo, P. B., Nwameme, A., Cole, H. V. S., Maya, E., Liu, M., et al. (2016). mHealth to train community health nurses in visual inspection with acetic acid for cervical cancer screening in Ghana. *Journal of Lower Genital Tract Disease, 20,* 239–242. https://doi. org/10.1097/LGT.0000000000000207.

Atkin, C. K., & Wallack, L. M. (1990). *Mass communication and public health: Complexities and conflicts.* Newbury Park: Sage Publications.

Atun, R. (2012). Health systems, systems thinking and innovation. *Health Policy and Planning, 27* (suppl 4), iv4–iv8. doi:10.1093/heapol/czs088.

Bajwa, M. (2014). mHealth security. *Pakistan Journal of Medical Sciences, 30*(4), 904.

Bakshi, A., Narasimhan, P., Li, J., Chernih, N., Ray, P. K., & MacIntyre, R. (2011). mHealth for the control of TB/HIV in developing countries. In *e-Health Networking Applications and Services (Healthcom), 2011 13th IEEE International Conference on* (pp. 9–14). IEEE.

Bullen, P. A. B. (2013). Operational challenges in the Cambodian mHealth revolution. *Journal of Mobile Technology in Medicine, 2*(2), 20–23.

Castelnuovo, G., Manzoni, G. M., Pietrabissa, G., Corti, S., Giusti, E. M., Molinari, E., et al. (2014). Obesity and outpatient rehabilitation using mobile technologies: The potential mHealth approach. *Frontiers in Psychology, 5,* 559.

Chang, L. W., Njie-Carr, V., Kalenge, S., Kelly, J. F., Bollinger, R. C., & Alamo-Talisuna, S. (2013). Perceptions and acceptability of mHealth interventions for improving patient care at a community-based HIV/AIDS clinic in Uganda: A mixed methods study. *AIDS Care, 25*(7), 874–880.

Chib, A. (2013). The promise and peril of mHealth in developing countries. *Mobile Media & Communication, 1*(1), 69–75.

Comstock, J. (2014, January 2). Samsung gets FDA clearance for S Health app. *Mobi Health News.* Retrieved from http://mobihealthnews.com/28387/samsung-gets-fda-clearance-for-s-health-app.

Cumiskey, K. M., & Hjorth, L. (2013). *Mobile media practices, presence and politics: The challenge of being seamlessly mobile.* New York: Routledge.

de Jongh, T., Gurol-Urganci, I., Vodopivec-Jamsek, V., Car, J., & Atun, R. (2012). Mobile phone messaging for facilitating self-management of long-term illnesses. *The Cochrane Database of Systematic Reviews, 12,* CD007459.

Droppert, H., & Bennett, S. (2015). Corporate social responsibility in global health: An exploratory study of multinational pharmaceutical firms. *Globalization and Health, 11*(15), 1–8. https://doi.org/10.1186/s12992-015-0100-5.

Dutta, M. J. (2005). Theory and practice in health communication campaigns: A critical interrogation. *Health Communication, 18*(2), 103–122.

Dutta, M. J. (2008). *Communicating health: A culture-centered approach.* London: Polity.

Dutta, M. J. (2011). *Communicating social change: Structure, culture, and agency.* New York: Routledge.

Dutta, M. J. (2015). *Neoliberal health organizing.* New York, NY: Routledge.

Dutta-Bergman, M. J. (2005). Theory and practice in health communication campaigns: A critical interrogation. *Health Communication, 18*(2), 103–122. https://doi.org/10.1207/s15327027hc1802_1.

Ericsson. (2008). *Ericsson and Apollo Hospitals to bring healthcare access to rural India [Press release].* Retrieved June 5 from https://www.ericsson.com/news/1225191.

Fiordelli, M., Diviani, N., & Schulz, P. J. (2013). Mapping mHealth research: A decade of evolution. *Journal of Medical Internet Research, 15*(5), e95.

Free, C., Phillips, G., Watson, L., Galli, L., Felix, L., Edwards, P., et al. (2013). The effectiveness of mobile-health technologies to improve health care service delivery processes: A systematic review and meta-analysis. *PLoS Medicine, 10,* e1001363. https://doi.org/10.1371/journal. pmed.1001363.

Gurman, T. A., Rubin, S. E., & Roess, A. A. (2012). Effectiveness of mHealth behavior change communication interventions in developing countries: A systematic review of the literature. *Journal of Health Communication, 17,* 82–104. https://doi.org/10.1080/10810730.2011. 649160.

Hall, C. S., Fottrell, E., Wilkinson, S., & Byass, P. (2014). Medicinska fakulteten, Epidemiologi och folkhälsovetenskap, Institutionen för folkhälsa och klinisk medicin. Assessing the impact of mHealth interventions in low- and middle-income countries: What has been shown to work? *Global Health Action, 7,* 25606–25612. https://doi.org/10.3402/gha.v7.25606.

Handford, R. (2012). Smart works with Philippines government on mHealth. *Mobile World Live.* Retrieved from July 2 http://www.mobileworldlive.com/latest-stories/smart-works-with-philippines-government-on-mhealth/.

Healthcare Asia. (2014). *Who's winning the $10.8bn Asian mHealth race?* Retrieved October 9 from http://healthcareasiamagazine.com/healthcare/feature/who%E2%80%99s-winning-108bn-asian-mhealth-race.

International Telecommunication Union. (2016). *ICT facts and figures 2016.* Retrieved from http://www.itu.int/en/ITU-D/Statistics/Pages/facts/default.aspx.

Istepanian, R., Laxminarayan, S., & Pattichis, C. S. (2006). *M-health: Emerging mobile health systems.* New York, NY: Springer Science + Business Media, Incorporated.

Jennings, L., Lee, N., Shore, D., Strohminger, N., Allison, B., Conserve, D. F., et al. (2016). U.S. minority homeless youth's access to and use of mobile phones: Implications for mHealth intervention design. *Journal of Health Communication, 21,* 725. https://doi.org/10.1080/10810730.2015.1103331.

Johns Hopkins Bloomberg School of Public Health. (2012). Mobile technology for health in rural Bangladesh. *The JiVita Journal.* Retrieved from jhsph.edu/research/centers-and-institutes/center-for-human-nutrition/research/jivita/journal/JivitaJournal08_mHealth_September%202012_compressed.pdf.

Kahn, J. G., Yang, J. S., & Kahn, J. S. (2010). 'Mobile' health needs and opportunities in developing countries. *Health Affairs, 29*(2), 252–258.

Kaplan, W. A. (2006). Can the ubiquitous power of mobile phones be used to improve health outcomes in developing countries? *Globalization and Health, 2,* 1–14.

Katz, R., Mesfin, T., & Barr, K. (2012). Lessons from a community-based mHealth diabetes self-management program: "It's not just about the cell phone". *Journal of Health Communication, 17*(Suppl. 1), 67–72. https://doi.org/10.1080/10810730.2012.650613.

Kay, M., Santos, J., & Takane, M. (2011). mHealth: New horizons for health through mobile technologies. *World Health Organization, 64*(7), 66–71.

Khan, N., Rasheed, S., Sharmin, T., Ahmed, T., Mahmood, S. S., Khatun, F., et al. (2015). Experience of using mHealth to link village doctors with physicians: Lessons from Chakaria, Bangladesh. *BMC Medical Informatics and Decision Making, 15,* 62. https://doi.org/10.1186/s12911-015-0188-9e17.

Khatun, F., Heywood, A. E., Ray, P. K., Bhuiya, A., & Liaw, S. (2016). Community readiness for adopting mHealth in rural Bangladesh: A qualitative exploration. *International Journal of Medical Informatics, 93,* 49–56. https://doi.org/10.1016/j.ijmedinf.2016.05.010.

Khokhar, A. (2009). Short text messages (SMS) as a reminder system for making working women from Delhi breast aware. *Asian Pacific Journal of Cancer Prevention, 10,* 319–322.

Kim, Y. (2010). *Building broadband: Strategies and policies for the developing world.* Washington, DC: World Bank Publications. https://doi.org/10.1596/978-0-8213-8419-0.

Labrique, A., Vasudevan, L., Chang, L. W., & Mehl, G. (2013). H_pe for mHealth: More "y" or "o" on the horizon? *International Journal of Medical Informatics, 82*(5), 467–469.

Levin, D. (2012). mHealth: Promise and pitfalls. *Frontiers of Health Services Management, 29,* 33–39.

Lupton, D. (1994). Toward the development of critical health communication praxis. *Health Communication, 6,* 55–67. https://doi.org/10.1207/s15327027hc0601_4.

Malvey, D., & Slovensky, D. J. (2014). *mHealth: Transforming healthcare.* New York, NY: Springer.

Manda, T. D., & Sanner, T. A. (2014). The mobile is part of a whole: Implementing and evaluating mHealth from an information infrastructure perspective. *International Journal of User-Driven Healthcare (IJUDH), 4,* 1–16. https://doi.org/10.4018/ijudh.2014010101.

McBride, C. M., & Rimer, B. K. (1999). Using the telephone to improve health behavior and health service delivery. *Patient Education and Counselling, 37,* 3–18.

Mechael, P. N. (2009). The case for mHealth in developing countries. *Innovations, 4,* 103–118.

mHealth Alliance. (2013). *Patient privacy in a mobile world: A framework to address privacy law issues in mobile health.* Retrieved from http://mhealthknowledge.org/resources/patient-privacy-mobile-world-framework-addresses-privacy-law-issues-mobile-health.

Nachega, J. B., Skinner, D., Jennings, L., Magidson, J. F., Altice, F. L., Burke, J. G., et al. (2016). Acceptability and feasibility of mHealth and community-based directly observed antiretroviral therapy to prevent mother-to-child HIV transmission in South African pregnant women under option B +: An exploratory study. *Patient Preference and Adherence, 10,* 683–690. https://doi.org/10.2147/PPA.S100002.

Norberg, M. M., Rooke, S. E., Albertella, L., Copeland, J., Kavanagh, D. J., & Lau, A. Y. (2015). The first mHealth app for managing cannabis use: Gauging its potential helpfulness. *Addictive Behaviors, Therapy and Rehabilitation, 3*(1).

Olla, P., & Shimskey, C. (2015). mHealth taxonomy: A literature survey of mobile health applications. *Health and Technology, 4,* 299–308. https://doi.org/10.1007/s12553-014-0093-8.

Pattichis, R. S. H., Istepanian, C. S., & Laxminarayan, S. (2006). Ubiquitous m-Health systems and the convergence towards 4G mobile technologies. In R. S. H. Istepanian, S. Laxminarayan, & C. S. Pattichis (Eds.), *M-Health: Emerging mobile health systems* (pp. 3–14). USA: Springer Science + Business Media Inc.

Pinnock, H., Slack, R., Pagliari, C., Price, D., & Sheikh, A. (2007). Understanding the potential role of mobile phone-based monitoring on asthma self-management: Qualitative study. *Clinical and Experimental Allergy, 37*(5), 794–802.

PLOS Medicine Editors. (2013). A reality checkpoint for mobile health: Three challenges to overcome. *PLoS Med, 10*(2), e1001395.

Post, L. A., Vaca, F. E., Doran, K. M., Luco, C., Naftilan, M., Dziura, J., et al. (2013). New media use by patients who are homeless: The potential of mHealth to build connectivity. *Journal of Medical Internet Research, 15*(9), e195.

PricewaterhouseCoopers. (2012). *Touching lives through mobile health: Assessment of the global market opportunity.* Retrieved from http://www.pwc.in/assets/pdfs/telecom/gsma-pwc_mhealth_report.pdf.

Qiang, C. Z., Yamamichi, M., Hausman, V., & Altman, D. (2011). *Mobile applications for the health sector.* World Bank. Retrieved from http://siteresources.worldbank.org/INFORMATIONANDCOMMUNICATIONANDTECHNOLOGIES/Resources/mHealth_report.pdf.

Rama, M., Béteille, T., Li, Y., Mitra, P. K., & Newman, J. L. (2014). *Addressing inequality in South Asia.* World Bank Publications.

Rhee, C. (2013). *Inequality in Asia and the Pacific: Trends, drivers and policy implications.* New York: Routledge.

Schnall, R., Rojas, M., Bakken, S., Brown, W., Carballo-Dieguez, A., Carry, M., et al. (2016). A user-centered model for designing consumer mobile health (mHealth) applications (apps). *Journal of Biomedical Informatics, 60,* 243–251.

Schweitzer, J., & Synowiec, C. (2012). The economics of eHealth and mHealth. *Journal of Health Communication, 17,* 73–81. https://doi.org/10.1080/10810730.2011.649158.

Shukla, S. N., & Sharma, J. K. (2016). Potential of mHealth to transform healthcare in India. *Journal of Health Management, 18*(3), 447–459.

Steinhubl, S. R., Muse, E. D., & Topol, E. J. (2013). Can mobile health technologies transform health care? *The Journal of the American Medical Association, 310*(22), 2395–2396.

Thomsen, S. C., Skinner, D., Toefy, Y., Esterhuizen, T., McCaul, M., Petzold, M., et al. (2016). Voice-message-based mHealth intervention to reduce postoperative penetrative sex in recipients of voluntary medical male circumcision in the Western Cape, South Africa: Protocol of a randomized controlled trial. *JMIR Research Protocols, 5*(3), e155. https://doi.org/10.2196/resprot.5958.

Tomlinson, M., Rotheram-Borus, M. J., Swartz, L., & Tsai, A. C. (2013). Scaling up mHealth: Where is the evidence? *PLoS Med, 10*(2), e1001382.

Watterson, J. L., Walsh, J., & Madeka, I. (2015). Using mHealth to improve usage of antenatal care, postnatal care, and immunization: A systematic review of the literature. *BioMed Research International, 2015*, 1–9. https://doi.org/10.1155/2015/153402.

White, A., Thomas, D. S. K., Ezeanochie, N., & Bull, S. (2016). Health worker mHealth utilization: A systematic review. *CIN: Computers Informatics, Nursing, 34*, 206–213. https://doi.org/10.1097/CIN.0000000000000231.

World Bank. (2008). *Global economic prospects 2008: Technology diffusion in the developing world*. Herndon: The World Bank. https://doi.org/10.1596/978-0-8213-7365-1.

World Health Organization. (2011). *mHealth: New horizons for health through mobile technologies*. Retrieved from http://www.who.int/goe/publications/goe_mhealth_web.pdf.

Zapata, D. B. (2016). Inayan/nga-ag and other indigenous codes: How the Applai and Bontok Igorot's indigeneity found its way into the mobile world. *Telematics and Informatics*. https://doi.org/10.1016/j.tele.2016.05.019.

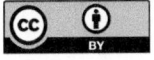

Chapter 7
Smart Health Facilitator: Chinese Consumers' Perceptions and Interpretations of Fitness Mobile Apps

Huan Chen

Abstract A phenomenological study was conducted to explore how Chinese consumers perceive fitness mobile apps in their everyday lives. Twenty in-depth interviews were used to collect data. Findings suggested that the meanings of mobile fitness apps are multidimensional, dialectical, and multilayered. On the positive side, mobile fitness apps embody control, empowerment, and networked individualism which assist Chinese consumers in achieving their fitness goals, maintaining healthy lifestyles, and enhancing the quality of their lives. On the negative side, mobile fitness apps have a constraining effect, geographically and temporally speaking. Some participants even linked fitness app use to their feelings of loneliness. Practical implications were offered to mobile fitness app companies and health organizations.

Keywords Fitness mobile app · Chinese consumer · Qualitative research

7.1 Introduction

According to eMarketer (Statista, 2016), there were more than 1 billion Chinese mobile phone users in 2015. The number of Chinese mobile Internet users has reached 695.3 million and 72.6% of the mobile Internet users in China live in cities (CNNIC, 2017). Many such consumers—especially Chinese urban consumers—are intentionally or unintentionally integrating their smartphones into their everyday fitness and health routines by way of mobile fitness apps. For example, Keep, one of the most popular fitness apps in China, has more than 30 million users (Dahl, 2016). Although data on mobile fitness apps use exists, to date no study has been conducted to examine how Chinese consumers perceive and experience those apps, and the broader social, and cultural changes these experiences may flag. Previous qualitative research on mHealth in China has focused on health education, chronic

H. Chen (✉)
College of Journalism and Communications, University of Florida, Gainesville, USA
e-mail: huanchen@jou.ufl.edu

© Asian Development Bank 2018
E. Baulch et al. (eds.), *mHealth Innovation in Asia*, Mobile Communication in Asia:
Local Insights, Global Implications, https://doi.org/10.1007/978-94-024-1251-2_7

disease management and texting for health, but not on more recent developments, such as smartphone-enabled health and fitness apps. Broader scholarship on fitness apps has been primarily quantitative and positivist in nature; little of the existing work on fitness apps explores their qualitative dimensions.

The current study is designed to fill this research gap. It not only extends existing scholarship but also holds important implications for fitness app development and for healthcare management. Its qualitative approach affords fitness apps developers with useful insights needed to tailor their products to Chinese consumers. It also holds the potential to inform Chinese healthcare organizations on how to use mobile fitness apps to help their patients manage their health and wellbeing.

7.2 Gaps in the Literature

A substantial body of scholarship dedicated to mHealth in China has begun to emerge in the recent years. This includes studies of health education, medication adherence, and appointment reminders (Corpman, 2013), the use of mobile technologies to extend health services to rural areas (Ni, Wu, Samples, & Shaw, 2014), and the use of mHealth for mental illness (Zhang, Song, & Bai, 2013). However, much of this research is yet to catch up with the rapid proliferation of smartphones across Asia. Therefore, little of this work focusses on social and cultural implications of fitness app use. Nor does the scholarship in fitness apps more broadly include much work on the qualitative dimensions of their use. Existing research on mobile fitness apps is dominated by quantitative work within a positivist framework of behavior change (Conroy, Yang, & Maher, 2014; West et al., 2012; Kranz et al., 2012; Chen & Pu, 2014; Millington, 2014; Lister, West, Cannon, Sax, & Brodegard, 2014). Conroy et al. (2014) found that the top ranked fitness mobile apps can be categorized as either educational or motivational, and the most common behavior change techniques used in those apps include providing information or demonstrating specific physical activities. West et al. (2012) examined the health and fitness mobile apps and found personal health and wellness, physical activity, and healthy eating apps to be the most represented categories. They studied the capacity of these apps to effect behavioral change and found that: (1) more than half of the apps are established upon predisposing factors which are primarily knowledge-based; (2) the most commonly used apps are those based upon enabling factors, such as teaching skills, tracking progress, or recording actual behavior; and (3) only few apps include reinforcing factors which are characterized by the provision of encouragement, evaluation, and the opportunity to interact with others.

Chen and Pu (2014) investigated the social incentives driving uses of mobile fitness apps and found that a mixture of cooperation and competition provides better social incentives than mere competition. Messages exchanged between participants cooperating with one another served to better motivate users than those exchanged among people competing with one another. Moreover, the more the users exchanged messages the better the results of their physical activities.

Millington (2014) qualitatively content analyzed eight prominent mobile fitness apps and found three major themes which are bettering the self, networked individualism, and mobility.

Studying the gamification of mobile fitness apps, Lister et al. (2014) found industry standards of effective gaming for fitness to be lacking. Stragier and Mechant (2013) surveyed consumers tweeting workouts activities which refers to the sharing of physical activities via social media such as Facebook and Twitter. A possible tweet of this would be "Just completed a 9.23 km run" or "Finished 30 min yoga practice today." They found that community identification, receiving feedback, and sharing information positively influence attitude toward tweeting workouts, which in turn has a positive effect on their tweeting workouts behaviors.

This chapter seeks to extend current work on fitness apps; I contend that qualitative research that enhances our understanding of users' perspectives is needed to better grasp some of the cultural and social implications of fitness apps' proliferation in recent years. The current study explores Chinese consumers' perceptions of fitness apps. It seeks to offer a rich description of mobile fitness apps from consumers' point of view, thereby providing important contextual information needed to bring research of mHealth in China up to date with recent developments, and to contribute a qualitative dimension to existing work on fitness apps. A thorough understanding of Chinese consumers' perceptions of fitness mobile apps also holds important implications for future app development and healthcare management.

7.3   Methodology

The question I address in this study is how Chinese consumers interpret mobile fitness apps as part of their everyday life. I used interpretative phenomenology analysis (IPA) to explore this question. IPA is a qualitative research method aimed at revealing the meanings a particular phenomenon holds for participants, and it involves the researcher interpreting the participants as they themselves interpret what is happening around them (Smith, Flowers, & Larkin, 2009). IPA has been widely applied in health research to explore a variety of topics (Smith, 1996; Fade, 2004; Brocki & Wearden, 2006). It is considered as a useful and valuable research method for understanding health care from the patient or service user perspective (Biggerstaff & Thompson, 2008).

According to App Annie (2016), the top fitness and health mobile apps in China include Keep, CoDoon, MiFit, Run, and Nike + Run Club, and indeed these apps emerge from the current study as significant to participants' fitness regimes. Since the majority of the smartphone users are living in urban areas (CIW, 2015), the study targeted Chinese urban consumers, of at least 18 years old, who owned a smartphone, and were current fitness app users. Purposive sampling and snowball sampling guided recruitment of participants. The criterion for sufficient sampling is saturation, that is, the point at which no new concepts and themes emerge

(Corbin & Strauss, 2008). In total, 20 participants (eight males and twelve females) were recruited and participated in the study. Their ages ranged from 18 to 70 years and their experience with mobile fitness apps ranged from 2 months to 4 years (Table 7.1).

In-depth interviews were used to collect data. The in-depth interview is the most commonly used method in phenomenological investigation (Moustakas, 1994; Thompson, Locander, & Pollio, 1990). It is a powerful qualitative method of phenomenological investigation because it "gives us the opportunity to step into the mind of another person, to see and experience the world as they do themselves" (McCracken, 1988, p. 9). It only sets broad parameters for the discussion, leaving participants free to tell their own stories. A loosely structured, discursive conversation is a good way to access participants' conscious experiences and allow their realities to emerge. Specifically, online in-depth interviews via WeChat were used to collect data. Previous research (Deakin & Wakefield, 2014) suggests that although there are benefits and drawbacks, online interviewing via social media messaging software can be useful to supplement face-to-face interviews. WeChat has a video chatting function. All the in-depth interviewers were conducted using video chatting. In this way, the researcher could interact with her participants and notice their nonverbal cues, just as in offline face-to-face interview situations. Each interview lasted approximately 30 min. To provide an accurate record of participants' comments, all the interviews were audio recorded and professionally transcribed.

Focused on the central phenomenon under investigation and broad research question, an interview guide was developed to reveal the meanings the participants constructed for mobile fitness apps and to initiate and facilitate conversations with participants. The main topics discussed during the conversations include participants' general workout routines, their selection and adoption of mobile fitness apps, their usage and experiences of mobile fitness apps, advantages and disadvantages of mobile fitness apps, and their suggestions for future improvement of mobile fitness apps. Following the emergent design tradition in qualitative research (Creswell, 2013), I changed and adjusted specific questions during each in-depth interview informed and guided by my participants' responses.

Four major themes emerged from the data set, which I discuss below. One theme refers to various ways in which the participants selected and adopted fitness apps, during the process they made decisions on which mobile apps to download either paid or free and to integrate them into their everyday workout routine. Such variations unfolded along the lines of singular use (use of one app) versus multiple use (downloading and use of multiple apps). Another referred to the various ways apps enabled people to control and order their lives. On the one hand, some participants spoke of their use of apps to motivate a life-changing fitness regime. On the other, others spoke of the limitations of apps' amenability to a variety of fitness practices. A third theme referred to people's different perceptions about the apps' capacities to improve their quality of life. Some participants talked about how using fitness apps improved their state of mind and general happiness, while others expressed concerns over becoming too dependent on the apps. A final theme referred to the

Table 7.1 Profile of participants

Name	Age	Gender	Education	Occupation	Apps	Length
Jean	39	Female	MA	Owner of a casual restaurant	My Asics, Adidas train and run, Connect, Run, Codoon	4 years
Christina	34	Female	MA	Public relations specialist	FitTime Keep Nike training	2 years
Linda	33	Female	MA	Teacher	Keep	4 months
Henry	38	Male	BS	IT technician	Codoon Run	4 years
Jade	35	Female	MA	Editor	TulipSport	2 years
Alpha	32	Male	BA	Salesman	Codoon Digital scale Keep	3 years
Lily	34	Female	BA	Director	动动	1 year
Peter	18	Male	High School	Undergraduate student	Keep	4 months
Wendy	19	Female	High School	Undergraduate student	Keep	2 months
Nancy	23	Female	BA	Graduate student	Fit time Body build up Insanity Nike + 轻+ 大姨妈	2 years
Sunny	53	Female	AA	Accountant	WeChat Health	6 months
Mandy	26	Female	BA	Account executive	Keep Nike + Codoon	5 months
Leo	70	Male	BA	Retired	WeChat Health Codoon	2 years
John	19	Male	High school	Undergraduate student	Nike training Keep	2 years
Tom	35	Male	BA	Graphic designer	Nike running and training Adidas Running and training Keep	3 years
Susan	26	Female	MA	Teacher	WeChat Health	6 months

(continued)

Table 7.1 (continued)

Name	Age	Gender	Education	Occupation	Apps	Length
Sam	21	Male	High school	Undergraduate student	Keep	9 months
Jenny	24	Female	BA	Secretary	Codoon Keep	1 year
Jolie	27	Female	MA	Teacher	FitTime Keep Nike running	2 years
Benny	34	Male	Ph.D.	Assistant professor	My Asics, Adidas train and run, Connect, Run, Codoon	1 and a half year

various capacities of apps to connect people to one another or, conversely, make them feel lonely. Some participants stated that they felt fitness apps did little to connect those seeking to take part in conventional team sports, such as basketball or football. Others enjoyed the online socializing that took place among those using a particular app.

7.4 Singular Versus Multiple Use

The interviews reveal participants selected and adopted mobile fitness apps in various ways. One group of people (n = 10) selected and downloaded one fitness app and used just that one app. A second group of people (n = 3) selected and downloaded multiple mobile fitness apps but used only one app; a third group (n = 7) selected, downloaded, and used multiple mobile fitness apps. The participants' fitness and health goals and knowledge of fitness and technology seemed to play a role in this selection and adoption process. In general, people with clear fitness goals have more knowledge of fitness and technology, and tended to choose and use multiple mobile fitness apps. Participants' level of comfort with mobile technologies was also a factor determining the number of apps they used as the following quotes from Sunny, Nancy, and Jean show:

> I only use WeChat Health to track my steps, and I don't use other mobile fitness apps. (R: Why not?) I feel that other mobile fitness apps are complicated and I don't have a strong fitness goal such as losing weight like others. … I know iPhone has a health app. But it requires too much personal information. I don't want to input too much of my information. I'm a little concerned. So I don't use it either (Sunny, female, 53, accountant).

> I tried a lot different mobile fitness apps. If I know there is a new app, I will download and try it. If I don't like it, I will then delete it. … The only app that I have been using for two years is the period tracking app called "大姨妈" (big aunt) (Nancy, female, 23, graduate student).

I use multiple mobile fitness apps in my daily life. I'm using My Asics, Adidas Train & Run, Connect, Run, and Codoon. You know, each of these apps performs different functions for me. My Asics tells me all the statistics of my health, like my heartbeat, sleep quality, my pulse, and so forth. Adidas Train & Run shows me all my running data. It not only tells me how long I run and tracks my running path. It also informs me about other specialized data such as my average pace, heart rate, average altitude and so forth (Jean, female, 39, owner of a casual restaurant).

Previous research revealed some personal and social incentives that may motivate consumers to use and experience fitness mobile apps (Chen & Pu, 2014; Millington, 2014). For instance, Chen and Pu (2014) emphasized the social incentives of competition and corporation while Millington (2014) focused on a broader personal incentive of bettering the self. The current study uncovers another important personal factor—the knowledge of fitness and technology as a possible motivational incentive for consumers to adopt mobile fitness apps. Compared to previous research (Chen & Pu, 2014; Millington, 2014), the incentive revealed in the current study is more self-oriented and specific, which brings some implications for both app developers and healthcare workers. One of the important implications is that app developers and healthcare workers need to take into account the various levels of technological literacy that exist among users when promoting and encouraging people to use mobile fitness apps. For example, app developers may design different versions of one mobile fitness app tailored to different user groups' needs. For users with little knowledge about fitness or lacking specific fitness goals, the version of the mobile app may embed more educational information of fitness knowledge and fitness goals to enhance users' literacy. Similarly, for users with rich knowledge of fitness and having specific fitness goals, the version of the mobile app may limit the educational content but add more advanced features and functions to help those users to meet their fitness needs in a more effective and efficient way. Healthcare workers should take patients' technology comfort level into consideration when recommending mobile fitness apps to their patients. For technology aversion patients, healthcare workers may show some easy-to-use mobile fitness apps to mitigate their stress and motivate them to try on those apps. By contrast, for technology savvy patients, healthcare workers should recommend mobile apps that better fit with their patients' healthy goals without worrying too much about technical issues they may encounter during their usage.

7.5 Apps that Afford Control Versus Apps that Constrain

According to the participants, the usage of mobile fitness apps on one hand offers them a sense of control; on the other hand, however, some participants felt that certain physical and geographical constraints inhered in fitness apps, and prevented them from using the apps in ways that fitted with their preferred fitness practices. The sense of control means better care of their health condition and body image, better time management, better knowledge of fitness, and ultimately a better life.

Many participants mentioned that mobile fitness apps helped them better track and monitor their daily physical activities, such as numbers of steps and duration of running time. Simply by seeing the numbers, they became more conscious of their health condition and are more motivated to work out and achieve their health and fitness goals. In addition, the participants also enjoyed the flexibility of mobile fitness apps that fits their everyday busy schedule. The participants also mentioned that mobile fitness apps helped to educate them about their health. Finally, they claimed that the apps facilitated their behavior change and formed a healthy life routine thus improving the quality of their lives. Henry, a 38-year-old IT technician, told the researcher that his workout and mobile fitness apps improved the quality of his life.

> It's a long story. You know, I'm an IT worker. I work long hours. It is a very stressful career. After I had my second child, my wife quit her job and became stay-at-home mom. I was the only bread winner. I felt much more stressed. That was a few years ago. At that time, I felt that my health condition was not very good. I wanted to sleep all the time and felt dizzy at 4 o'clock in the afternoon. I realized I have to change to make my life better. So I downloaded Codoon and started running. I was an amateur runner back then. I had no knowledge about running. I run a short distance every day and Codoon tracked my running records. After running for a while, I felt that my condition improved. I joined the online community of Codoon and know many running lovers there. We shared our running experiences, communicated, and supported each other. My knowledge of running increased through those online exchanges. With my friends' encouragement, I decided to run a marathon. I first ran a mini marathon, and then 5 km marathon to 10 km marathon. Now I participate in marathon every year. During the process, I felt that I need more specialized and professional app. Therefore I downloaded Nike Running and later bought Garmin watch. ... Running not only improved my health condition but also helped with my mind. A few years ago, I didn't read books. I felt that I read too slow and can never finish reading a book. After my health condition is getting better, my brain seems improved as well. Now I'm reading much faster and I try to read a book every month. Since I benefited from my running experiences, I also encouraged my wife to run. Now, she runs an hour every evening after putting our children into bed. ... In summary, I'd say that running has changed my life and improved the quality of my life (Henry, male, 38, IT technician).

As is evident from the above quote, mobile fitness apps afford users a sense of control over their bodies and lives. Previous research suggests that one of the most important claimed benefits of mobile fitness apps is enabling clear, quantifiable, improvements in personal health (Millington, 2014). Findings of the current study offered a detailed, rich, in-depth, and thick description of this claimed benefit from consumers' own perspective thus materializing and concretizing the concept in the cultural context of China.

While some participants deemed mobile fitness apps to enable them to better manage their lives, other spoke of apps' limited capacity to fit with and enhance a diverse range of fitness practices. Some participants mentioned that the mobile fitness apps limited their outdoor activities. They pointed out that they have to watch videos and follow instructors via certain mobile fitness apps. Therefore, they can only exercise in indoor spaces such as their own houses or apartments. Other participants indicated that their workouts were constrained by limited options on mobile fitness apps. For example, some mobile fitness apps only offer a certain number of exercises videos and others can only track certain kinds of workouts. Sam, a 21-year-old undergraduate student, and Wendy, a 19-year-old freshman both talked about the limitations of mobile fitness apps.

> I can only use mobile fitness apps in my house or my dorm. I have to follow the videos via the apps. Sometimes, the videos require some equipment which I don't have at home. … How to say, I work out not just for exercise but also to relax and have fun which I believe the mobile fitness app cannot offer to me (Sam, male, 21, undergraduate student).

> I don't like Keep. (R: Why?) When I use Keep, I can only use it at home by myself. I'd like to go to gym. In gym, I can work out, talk to my friends, and listen to music. In addition, there are also professional trainers in the gym to help me with my training, When I use Keep, I can only figure out the skills by myself (Wendy, female, 19, undergraduate student).

Similar to previous research, the current study found that the perceived usefulness and benefits (Deng, 2013) as well as facilitating conditions (Zhang et al., 2013) are shaping Chinese consumers' evaluation of mobile fitness apps. Specifically, according to the participants, as revealed by the current study, the perceived usefulness and benefits means better care of their health condition and body image, better time management, better knowledge of fitness, and ultimately a better life while the facilitating condition refers to the overall affordance enabled by functionality of mobile fitness apps. In addition, the current study further revealed "control" as an essential factor that may facilitate Chinese consumers' usage and experience of mobile fitness apps. Thus, companies and healthcare workers should try to enhance consumers' sense or perceived sense of control when promoting and encouraging people to use mobile fitness apps.

7.6 Improved Quality of Life Versus Overdependence

Participants not only spoke of how the usage of mobile fitness apps helped them to lose weight, keep fit, and look better but also of the sense of empowerment that came from the improvement of their quality of life. They claimed that using mobile fitness apps challenged them, energized them, and helped them to gain mental strength. They also talked about how mobile fitness apps facilitated new kinds of social interactions. Leo, a 70-year-old retiree, discussed how exercise and mobile fitness apps helped him to live a better life.

> After I retired, I have much more time to exercise and to achieve some fitness goals. … Ten years ago, when I went to Grand Canyon and walked two hours, I felt exhausted. Last year, when I went to Los Glaciares National Park I walked the whole afternoon about 10 km and didn't feel very tired. … I downloaded Codoon a couple of years ago. I saw my friend shared his walking statistics on WeChat moments. I was curious. So I asked him. He told me it was a mobile fitness app. So I downloaded it as well. (R: How does Codoon perform a role in your everyday workout routine?) You know, the Codoon could record the duration of your walk and track the routes of your walk. You can share the information on your WeChat. Since many of my friends are using Codoon, we monitor and support each other.

Sometimes, we will communicate with each other about our workout experiences on WeChat. ... Well, mobile fitness apps helped me to achieve my goal which is live a better life every day (Leo, male, 70, retiree).

While applauding the advantages of mobile fitness apps, the participants also showed concerns regarding the negative side of this new type of technology. In particular, the participants expressed their concerns about the possibility of overdependence on the mobile fitness app, and how that may limit their freewill and hinder that independence.

You know, I had my daughter three months ago. I need to lose weight quickly. So I downloaded Keep and used it everyday. Now I feel that I have to have Keep to guide my workouts. Without using it, I don't want to budge my body. So I'm wondering if I'm too dependent on it (Mandy, female, 26).

Previous literature on both mHealth and mobile fitness apps mainly focuses on analysis of services and apps (Conroy et al., 2014; West et al., 2012) or consumers' cognitive and attitudinal evaluation of those services and apps (Deng, 2013; Zhang et al., 2013). Although a couple of previous studies (Corpman, 2013; Li et al., 2014) discussed some societal and environmental conditions of mHealth penetration in the context of China, the current study supplemented the previous literature by uncovering the possible societal consequences of mobile fitness apps from the perspectives of Chinese consumers.

7.7 Loneliness Versus Belonging

The participants expressed differing opinions as to whether the usage of mobile fitness apps alienates people from their social groups, or whether it connects them to online communities, enhancing their sense of belonging. Some participants indicated that the mobile fitness app makes them feel lonely because they used it to exercise alone. For example, when Peter, a 19-year-old engineer undergraduate student, was asked about his mobile fitness apps usage experiences, he spoke of his feeling of loneliness when using the mobile fitness apps. Similarly, Wendy, a 19-year-old food science undergraduate student also described a sense of alienation when using the mobile fitness app of Keep using her experiences of gym workouts as a reference.

I feel lonely (when using mobile fitness apps), you know. I like playing basketball, soccer or badminton with my friends. Even for running, I'd like to run with my friends in the field on campus. We are having fun together. I don't like exercising just by myself. It makes me feel lonely (Peter, male, 19, undergraduate).

I sometimes use Keep. But I prefer to go to the gym if it is possible. Using Keep by myself makes me feeling alienated, you know. You work out by yourself in a limited space. ... When you go to gym, you can see many people working out with you. I also enjoy the loud music in the gym (Wendy, female, 19, undergraduate).

By contrast, some participants believed that the mobile fitness apps provide a portal for them to connect with like-minded consumers thus fostering a sense of belongingness and togetherness. For instance, Jade, an editor in a publishing house, vividly described how mobile fitness apps connect her with running mates and later they formed a closed social media group to communicate and support each other.

> I'm using TulipSports …Because I shared my running statistics on my WeChat moments via TulipSports, one of my friends introduced me to a closed WeChat group formed by running lovers. At the beginning, this WeChat group was established by a few Tsing Hua university graduates. It is a closed social media group. You can join it only by invitation. Because of this, the group members are relatively upscale. However, the group is very active. People communicate and socialize online all the time. Basically, they use numbers to socialize. You need to check in everyday by telling people how long you've run, swim, or ride. Based on the statistics people submit, there is a daily rank on the first page of the group. It is very interesting to see people compete with each other to be honored on the first page (Jade, female, 35, editor).

Previous research on mHealth and mobile fitness apps investigated the role mHealth services play in interventions to address mental illness (Li et al., 2014; Stragier & Mechant, 2013; Chen & Pu, 2014). The current study engages this work by highlighting some of the novel dimensions of the link between mobile technologies and mental wellbeing. Above we see how people not only perceive fitness apps as technologies that enable or constrain their ability to maintain fit and healthy bodies, but also affect their ability to be social. Some interviewees consider fitness apps to impede on the social, but others consider them to enhance it. The social aspect of fitness apps is important for apps developers and health services to take into account. As these interviews with users show, the social affordances of fitness apps depend on the user, highlighting the difficulty of ascertaining a known social impact of any one fitness app. The various responses recorded above highlight the importance of trialing particular fitness apps in any endeavor to provoke behavioral change around fitness practices in a given population.

7.8 Conclusion

This study explored Chinese consumers' understandings of mobile fitness apps. The study uncovered four major themes with regard to the meanings that the participants constructed for mobile fitness apps. The study has several important scholarly implications. First, it revealed the selection and adoption of mobile fitness apps to be a complex and dynamic process. Similar to the general adoption of mHealth (Deng, 2013; Zhang et al., 2013), Chinese consumers' selection and adoption seems to be influenced by perceived usefulness and benefits, external cues, and subjective norms. In addition, the study uncovered a number of individual factors that shape the selection and adoption process such as fitness goals, fitness knowledge, technology knowledge, and comfortable level with technology.

As an interpretative phenomenological study, one of the most important contributions of the current study is to reveal the lived meanings of mobile fitness apps in the lifeworld of Chinese consumers. Findings of the study suggested that the meanings of mobile fitness apps are multidimensional, dialectical, and multilayered. On the positive side, mobile fitness apps embody control, empowerment, and networked individualism which assist Chinese consumers in achieving their fitness goals, maintaining healthy lifestyles, and enhancing the quality of their lives. On the negative side, mobile fitness apps have a constraining effect, geographically and temporally speaking. Some participants even linked fitness app use to their feelings of loneliness.

The current study also has several practical implications. It offers valuable information for mobile fitness apps companies to better design their products. For example, based on the findings of the study, app developers may consider including and/or enhancing the functions of setting goals, disseminating educational information, and building fitness-themed online communities. When designing marketing communication campaigns and messages, the companies should emphasize how their products could help Chinese consumers to enhance control, gain empowerment, and feel as connected individuals.

The study also offers useful insights for healthcare organizations to use mobile fitness apps to help their patients to better manage their health and live a healthier life. For example, healthcare professionals should encourage their patients to adopt mobile fitness apps and increase the frequency of their daily usage of those apps. Healthcare professionals could also emphasize the individual, social, and cultural benefits of the usage of mobile fitness apps. In particular, the physicians should reinforce the message that the mobile fitness apps could help their patient to achieve a better health condition thus living a better life.

Several limitations should be noted. This research provided a snapshot in time of a dynamic phenomenon. Participants' interpretations are culturally contextualized and bound to be dynamic, changing as cultural meanings shift. Longitudinal data could provide additional insights into the interpersonal dynamics and microcultural characteristics of users' lifeworlds regarding this particular phenomenon. This study focused on Chinese consumers' interpretation of mobile fitness apps. Although the recruited participants are diverse in terms of demographics, the complexity and dynamics of the population mean that the collected data may not be able to reflect nuances and multiplicity of the rich meanings. For example, many of the participants in the current study are from big cities. Chinese users from small cities may have different interpretations and emphasize different aspects than those from the metropolitan areas. Future research may recruit a more diverse sample to reveal those nuances and dynamics. Furthermore, the mobile fitness app has gained popularity and penetrated different socioeconomic layers, and the user structure is becoming more diverse. Studies designed to explore the dynamics and variations among subcultures and subgroups of mobile fitness apps users should enrich our understanding of this particular phenomenon.

References

AppAnnie. (2016, November 2). *Top apps on iOS store, China, overall.* Retrieved from https://www.appannie.com/apps/ios/top/china/overall/iphone/.

Biggerstaff, D., & Thompson, A. R. (2008). Interpretative phenomenological analysis (IPA): A qualitative methodology of choice in healthcare research. *Qualitative Research in Psychology, 5*(3), 214–224. https://doi.org/10.1080/14780880802314304.

Brocki, J., & Wearden, A. (2006). A critical evaluation of the use of interpretative phenomenological analysis (IPA) in health psychology. *Psychology and Health, 21*(1), 87–108. https://doi.org/10.1080/14768320500230185.

Chen, Y., & Pu, P. (2014). *HealthyTogether: Exploring social incentives for mobile fitness applications.* Paper presented at Second International Symposium of Chinese CHI (Chinese CHI 2014), April 26–27 2014, Toronto, Ontario, Canada. Retrieved from http://chchi2014.icachi.org/.

CIW team. (2015, October 12). *China smartphone penetration rate to reach 38.6% in 2015.* Retrieved from http://www.chinainternetwatch.com/14941/urban-smartphone-users-half-new-equipment-next-year/#ixzz4jFplMOZW.

CNNIC. (2017, January). *Chinese internet development report.* Retrieved from http://www.cnnic.cn/hlwfzyj/hlwxzbg/hlwtjbg/201701/P020170123364672657408.pdf.

Conroy, D. E., Yang, C. H., & Maher, J. P. (2014). Behavior change techniques in top-ranked mobile apps for physical activity. *American Journal of Preventive Medicine, 46*(6), 649–652.

Corbin, J., & Strauss, A. (2008). *Basics of qualitative research* (3rd ed.). Thousand Oaks, CA: Sage.

Corpman, D. (2013). Mobile health in China: A review of research and programs in medical care, health education, and public health. *Journal of Health Communication, 18,* 1345–1367.

Creswell, J. W. (2013). *Qualitative inquiry and research design: Choosing among five approaches* (3rd ed.). Washington, DC: Sage.

Dahl, J. (2016, May 22). Why VCs are putting their bets in Chinese fitness startups. *Forbes.* Retrieved from http://www.forbes.com/sites/jordyndahl/2016/05/22/why-vcs-are-putting-their-bets-in-chinese-fitness-startups/#7218bcf25bbd.

Deakin, H., & Wakefield, K. (2014). Skype interviewing: Reflections of two PhD researchers. *Qualitative Research, 14,* 603–616.

Deng, Z. (2013). Understanding public users' adoption of mobile health service. *International Journal of Mobile Communication, 11*(4), 351–373.

Fade, S. (2004). Using interpretative phenomenological analysis for public health nutrition and dietetic research: A practical guide. *Proceedings of the Nutrition Society, 63*(4), 647–653.

Kranz, M., Möller, B., Hammerlac, N., Diewald, S., Plötz, T., Olivier, P., et al. (2012). The mobile fitness coach: Towards individualized skill assessment using personalized mobile devices. *Persuasive and Mobile Computing.* https://doi.org/10.1016/j.pmcj.2012.06.002.

Li, H., Zhang, T., Chi, H., Chen, Y., Li, Y., & Wang, J. (2014). Mobile health in China: Current status and future development. *Asian Journal of Psychology, 10,* 101–104.

Lister, C., West, J. H., Cannon, B., Sax, T., & Brodegard, B. (2014). Just a fad? Gamification in health and fitness apps. *JMIR Serious Games, 2*(2). doi:10.2196/games.3413.

McCracken, G. (1988). *The long interview.* Newbury Park, CA: Sage.

Millington, B. (2014). Smartphone apps and the mobile privatization of health and fitness. *Critical Studies in Media Communication, 31*(5), 479–493.

Moustakas, C. (1994). *Phenomenological research methods.* Thousand Oaks, CA: Sage.

Ni, Z., Wu, B., Samples, C., & Shaw, R. J. (2014). Mobile technology for health care in rural China. *International Journal of Nursing Science,* 323–324.

Smith, J. A. (1996). Beyond the divide between cognition and discourse: Using interpretative phenomenological analysis in health psychology. *Psychology & Health, 11*(2), 261–271.

Smith, J., Flowers, P., & Larkin, M. (2009). *Interpretative phenomenological analysis: Theory, method and research.* Los Angeles, CA: Sage.

Statista. (2016). *Number of mobile phone users in China from 2013 to 2019*. Retrieved from http://www.statista.com/statistics/233291/forecast-of-mobile-phone-users-in-china/.

Stragier, J., & Mechant, P. (2013). Mobile fitness apps for promoting physical activity on Twitter: The #RunKeeper case. In *Proceedings of the Etmaal Van De Communicatiewetenschappen, Paper 67* (pp. 1–8). Rotterdam, The Netherlands. Retrieved from https://biblio.ugent.be/publication/3129098/file/3153471.pdf.

Thompson, C. J., Locander, W. B., & Pollio, H. R. (1990). The lived meaning of free choice: An existential-phenomenological description of everyday consumer experiences of contemporary married women. *Journal of Consumer Research, 17,* 346–361.

West, J. H., Hall, C. P., Hanson, C. L., Barnes, M. B., Giraud-Carrier, C., & Barrett, J. (2012). There's an app for that: Content analysis of paid health and fitness apps. *Journal of Medical Internet Research, 14*(3), 72–84.

Zhang, J., Song, Y. L., & Bai, C. X. (2013). MIOTIC study: A prospective, multicenter, randomized study to evaluate the long-term efficacy of mobile phone-based Internet of Things in the management of patients with stable COPD. *International Journal of Chronic Obstructive Pulmonary Disease, 8,* 433–438. https://doi.org/10.2147/COPD.S50205.

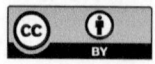

Chapter 8
Afterword: Reflections on a Decade of mHealth Innovation in Asia

Arul Chib

The role of mobile phones in healthcare improvement in Asia, particularly in resource-constrained contexts, is a significant topic, and there has long been a need for quality research to develop the field regionally. In this pursuit, this volume is a timely contribution, focusing our shared interests on the importance of sociocultural influences on the adoption, appropriation, and impact of varied mobile affordances on health. This is a timely tome, particularly considering a personal trajectory of research—it is a decade since the publication of our first paper on Indonesian midwives and mobiles post-tsunami (Chib, Lwin, Ang, & Santosa, 2008), and half a decade since I summarized the benefits of, and barriers to, mHealth impact in developing countries (Chib, 2013), culminating in a call for application of contextual and critical conceptualization, methodological plurality, and expansion of the evidence base. As many scholars in this volume present evidence in response to those projections made, it seems fitting that this concluding chapter respond to their contributions.

It is obvious that we need to interrogate the existing literature, theories utilized, assumptions made, and the evidence available. In the past decade, there has been a spate of review studies in mHealth (Blynn & Aubuchon, 2009; Fjeldsoe, Marshall, & Miller, 2009; Fry & Neff, 2009; Gurol-Urganci, de Jongh, Vodopivec-Jamsek, Car, & Atun, 2012; Klasnja & Pratt, 2012; Mechael et al., 2010; Patrick, Griswold, Raab, & Intille, 2008; Tomlinson, Rotheram-Borus, Swartz, & Tsai, 2013). More recently, the attention of mHealth reviews has shifted gradually toward developing countries (Agarwal, Perry, Long, & Labrique, 2015; Chib, van Velthoven, & Car, 2014; Deglise, Suggs, & Odermatt, 2012), with two of the four most-read studies in the Journal of Health Communication concerning mHealth (Gurman, Rubin, & Roess, 2012; Higgs, et al., 2014). A common refrain, echoed by the editors of this volume, in this range of review studies is the lack of rigorous evidence, particularly

A. Chib (✉)
Nanyang Technological University, Singapore, Singapore
e-mail: arulchib@ntu.edu.sg

© Asian Development Bank 2018
E. Baulch et al. (eds.), *mHealth Innovation in Asia*, Mobile Communication in Asia:
Local Insights, Global Implications, https://doi.org/10.1007/978-94-024-1251-2_8

in scaling pilot projects, usually program interventions conducted on small samples, to general populations. It is worthwhile to refrain on commenting on whether this volume addresses this research gap till we have reflected on the broader objectives strived for.

This manuscript provides a timely perspective within which to situate future developments for the use of mobile phones by healthcare service providers in resource-constrained contexts. The contributors to this volume present a range of studies based on empirical evidence from a range of Asian contexts. It is debatable whether any individual study provides substantive and irrefutable scientific evidence for mHealth impact, or an individual policy recommendation for mobile phone use (or a ban) within the formal healthcare system. However, taken as a whole, the volume can inform the complexity of policy development and enforcement, particularly illustrating the wide variety of sociocultural contexts encountered across communities in Asia. To provide an over-arching frame, this concluding chapter examines and interrogates the studies in the context of what appears to be the organic growth of mobile phone praxis in Asia. It is within this context that this concluding chapter will amplify the learnings from these current chapters versus a decade-long established trajectory of research, focusing on the sociocultural implications for the introduction, adoption, appropriation, and impact of mHealth for vulnerable communities in Asia.

Before we focus on the organic adoption and usage of mobile, we need to acknowledge the techno-deterministic framing of mobile phone use in planned interventions. Dutta, Kaur-Gill, Tan, and Lam present a critique of market- and state-driven logics of top-down mHealth interventions in Chap. 6. The culture-centered approach emphasized in this chapter promotes a critical perspective toward the implementation of mHealth projects in Asia, particularly hard to reach communities. The authors argue that the effects of mHealth are heavily dependent on the community in which the technology is deployed, with different environments and contexts leading to different outcomes. They identify a number of factors, similar to those stated by Evans, Bhatt, and Sharma in Chap. 3, including the problems faced by hard to reach communities where literacy and income levels are low, and traditional cultural barriers such as static gender roles are prevalent, thus impeding the adoption and growth of mHealth technologies. These authors propose a checklist for future mHealth programs run in low- and middle-income countries to overcome challenges and maximize effectiveness.

Evans et al. (see Chap. 3) develop a framework based on nine key components. At the technical level, tools have to be sustainable and feasible within the available infrastructure; hardware has to be context-appropriate, familiar and easily available to locals; and tool design has to be user-centered. At the organizational level, partnerships between the government and various enterprises will help establish a stable ecosystem for mHealth; the cooperation of the government through policies will support the integration of mHealth tools into the larger healthcare system. mHealth programs need to be financially sustainable through government support or other means, and use equipment that are cost-effective. In doing so, these authors reiterate prior categorizations of success factors in the field, such as the

Technology-Community-Management (TCM) model. The TCM model comprises the three intersects of technical factors, project management, and community participation for sustainable and successful mHealth interventions (Chib, Wilkin, & Hoefman, 2013). Especially relevant for this volume, the extended TCM model adds a vulnerability lens, arguing that sociocultural, informational, economic, and individual factors act as barriers.

Importantly, addressing vulnerable communities across Asia, Dutta et al. (Chap. 6) direct a critical lens on issues of power within mHealth. There is little doubt, despite our calls to strive for interdisciplinary collaborations, that the pendulum of mHealth research has swung in the direction of market-based interventions, with laboratory-based experiments and public health program interventions rife in the field. While these authors reiterate the intent of calls for future research to "examine potential shifts in power relationships caused by the introduction and adoption of mobile technologies in healthcare systems, and the extent and the limitations of their impact" (Chib, 2013, p. 5), they nonetheless limit the critical lens to state-driven and market-based mHealth programs. This volume provides a rich resource to investigate "the fissures that mobile systems implementation can introduce into the existing social-cultural hierarchies" (Chib, 2013, p. 5). There is much to be learnt from the organic adoption and appropriation of mobile technologies by communities in resource-constrained environments, particularly those most vulnerable. It is toward these issues that this chapter next turns, framing the contributions within the sociocultural, informational, economic, and individual vulnerabilities identified in the extended TCM model (Chib et al., 2013).

In Chap. 4, Pitaloka, investigating communicative practices related to diabetes among rural women in Java, Indonesia, found that many people in rural populations do not possess a smartphone and therefore cannot access relevant information. Similarly, utilizing a communicative ecologies framework in Chap. 5, Watkins and Baulch found two participants isolated from ongoing conversation within an HIV/AIDS network due to lack of the BlackBerry Messenger app, despite noting that in major regions of Indonesia, the required telecommunications infrastructure is present, with access to mobile phones and cellular networks not an issue. It is worth noting the multi-pronged nature of mHealth, with infrastructural challenges not limited to mere provision of communication networks and devices, but applicable to elements across the entire healthcare provision system. Watkins and Baulch (Chap. 5) found that medical supply issues and graft influenced the ability of community healthcare workers (CHWs) to keep their clients on ART (antiretroviral therapy) medication. These authors reiterate established facts within the literature related to economic and infrastructural challenges that are necessary to overcome before mHealth effectiveness can be brought to fruition in resource-constrained countries.

It is worth noting that with the relative ubiquity of mobile phones globally, as noted by the volume editors, that uneven technological infrastructure may not be the key barrier to mHealth success rates in the future; rather sociocultural factors may be a key concern when translating the usage of mobile technologies into positive health outcomes. Even in the case of provision of the requisite technological infrastructure by program managers in developing countries, individual resistance to change occurs. In Chap. 2, Tariq and Durrani interviewed female CHWs, who collect patients' health data via mHealth monitoring solutions developed to enhance antenatal care in rural populations in Pakistan. These lady health workers work at the frontline (margins) of the formal healthcare system, making healthcare accessible to communities that lack the infrastructure and resources for more advanced services. Despite providing the CHWs with the data entry module as a means to ease data collection on the spot, they mostly used the mHealth application only in the latter part of the day, keying in data from their paper-based records. This defeated the purpose of the mobile application, which was intended for on-the-fly collection of patient data, and interaction with specialists. Watkins and Baulch (Chap. 5), studying how community health workers integrated personal mobile devices into their work with HIV/AIDS patients, too point out that, CHWs preferred traditional methods of data collection and communication to mHealth solutions. Most stakeholders within the healthcare systems, including nongovernmental organizations, health institutions and individual health workers, had not integrated mHealth tools, continuing to prefer paper records, with the result that few of them had transitioned to the digital systems. Given these examples, we next need to examine the sociocultural considerations that limit structural transformation, rather than merely studying individual behavior change. The chapter next turns our attention to specific illustrations from the contributors.

Tariq and Durrani (Chap. 2) state the importance of communication in the development of mHealth apps, proposing a framework of strategies that advocate making device choices that are contextually sensitive. Within the frame of sociocultural vulnerabilities, the chapter provides examples of the intersections of marginalization that *khatoon* community health workers face in the socio-structural hierarchy of Pakistani society. Intersectionality theory (Crenshaw, 1989) discusses the dynamic, multifaceted, and contextually (historical and sociocultural) situated experience of women, illustrated in this case by oppression along the lines of class and gender. The case study describes age as significant factor for adoption and continued usage of the mobile device, with younger CHWs both more likely to access (and own) mobile phones and have the requisite digital literacy for productive use. The constrained patriarchal environment included disapproving fathers, untrustworthy male relatives (both their own and those of their female patients), and competing domestic duties. We can begin to unpack the intersections of oppression that influence (non-) adoption and (lack of) productive usage of the introduced mobile intervention.

We know that the layering of a supposedly neutral socio-technical infrastructure on top of an existing sociocultural context embedded with complex and biased power relationships creates considerable tensions (Chib, 2013). An SMS-based mHealth program intervention, delivered via an HIV/AIDS quiz in Uganda, was found to have created complications for vulnerable rural women (Chib, Wilkin, Leow, Hoefman, & van Bejima, 2012). The program failed to address economic vulnerabilities (low access and ownership of mobile phones), informational vulnerabilities (illiteracy and lack of knowledge about HIV testing compounded by testing information only being relayed to those with correct answers), and individual vulnerabilities (fear of being identified as HIV-positive). Requiring information about the HIV status of one's partner was compounded by the cultural communicative practice of shared mobile phone usage, creating a sociocultural vulnerability for women residing in deeply patriarchal societies, and rendering the program as potentially harmful as opposed to beneficial. The Pakistani case study (Chap. 2) conjectures that mediated interpersonal and mass media based campaigns be employed as micro- and macro-communicative strategies, but would gain considerable credibility if these recommendations were to be supported with empirical evidence linking these strategies to the sociocultural vulnerabilities presented. Further, these recommendations could be considerably strengthened were the analysis to be based on deliberation of the impact of the performance indicators identified. We can commend the attempt to utilize methodological pluralities to address the sensitive sociocultural issues identified. The relative strength of these communication tools (organic mobile-based strategies of individual actors vs. planned interventions, whether mobile-based or delivered via traditional mass media) can, allied with sophisticated and rigorous analysis, certainly provide context to policymakers.

The case studies from Indonesia and China provide us a rich evidence base to discuss sociocultural contexts across a number of dimensions. First, I shall continue to develop the particular dimension of gender as a key sociocultural dimension in Asia, elaborating on the patriarchal constraints identified. However, rather than merely considering this a barrier to the successful translation of mHealth introduction to public health outcomes, I advance the notion of technology appropriation as both a determinant of success (as articulated in health indicators) as well as a social outcome. Second, when arguing for the importance of sociocultural context, it is equally important to advance theoretical frames that are themselves driven from the ground up. To do so, I situate the learnings from the volume chapters within existing literature in the mHealth field.

First, it is hardly a coincidence that multiple chapters encounter the issue of gender inequality as a determinant of mHealth success. In particular, in Chap. 4, Pitaloka situates diabetes management via mobile communication within the context of gender empowerment and autonomy. In this case study, diabetic women in two rural Javanese villages have taken to using SMS as an alternative to diabetes apps, communicating with local health providers through their mobile phones, calling or texting them for help and advice regarding their health conditions, and receiving self-care reminders. As a consequence, texting seems to have become a practice and routine for diabetic self-management.

It is worth noting that agency and autonomy are complex phenomenon, and contested terms, in relation to gender and empowerment, thus require sensitive and meticulous elaboration (Nguyen, Chib, & Mahalingam, 2017). Pitaloka suggests that beyond traditional domestic roles, rural Javanese women, being petty traders, gain self-reliance as financial managers for the family. In addition, these women actively engage in public matters, particularly those related to religion. This vision of gender autonomy is interesting as mobile communicative practices reveal usage mediated by males, alongside a reinforcement of traditional gender roles amid structural inequalities. Despite claiming financial control, the women report being bought phones by their male children, feeling *pekewuh* or discomfort when using the phone due to perceived neglect of domestic duties, and feeling *sungkan* or shame when contacting the *mantri* or doctor, perceived as having higher social status. Such attitudes and behavior, both internalized and enacted, seem at odds with diabetes self-management, a far from trivial concern. This is not the only illustration—it is worth noting the active gender discrimination and low social status of Pakistani lady healthcare workers reported by Tariq and Durrani (Chap. 2) which inhibit the acceptance of mHealth solutions.

It would be interesting to analyze whether communicative behaviors merely indicate inhibited agency and autonomy or whether these tools can simultaneously produce resistance and negotiation in response to established sociocultural inequalities (Nguyen et al., 2017). In Chap. 4, Pitaloka regards text messages as communicative practices that create an alternative space for negotiation. This case echoes the dialectic negotiations via mobile communicative practices (including hiding and sharing) that midwives in Aceh Besar employed to develop a nascent gender consciousness in relation to their social positionalities (Chib & Chen, 2011). Like the Acehnese midwives, Javanese diabetics engaged in culturally appropriate communicative practices of restraint in purchase and usage of mobile phones, often mediating both these practices via males, allowing them to enact agency while minimizing possible social repercussions by upholding the unequal social order. This suggests that mHealth programs and practices then require evaluation beyond the immediate objectives of improved health outcomes, to encompass the broader range of social structural change that occurs simultaneously, particularly in the area of power inequality.

A final note concerns the hegemonic practice of solely applying theories, regardless of appropriate application, developed in, and in relation to, Western frames and contexts, which does the cultural heritage of Asian communities, and Asian researchers, a disservice. I discuss the importance of the development and advancement of culturally contextualized theoretical frames for mHealth in Asia, as Asian scholars find few opportunities to substantially contribute to original theory. Certainly theory requires generalizability from specific contexts to others, but should also shed light on and glean insights from them. As described earlier, the chapter by Pitaloka (Chap. 4) provides us a range of sociocultural norms such as *pekewuh* and *sungkan* that advance our understanding of the constraints facing Javanese women. Given the spate of mHealth studies concentrating on SMS (see Cole-Lewis & Kershaw, 2010; Deglise et al., 2012; Guy et al., 2012; Krishna, Boren, & Balas, 2009), it would be interesting to see how the Indonesian examples could inform (generalize to) the broader field.

In Chap. 5, Watkins and Baulch find that participants prefer face-to-face encounters to mediated communication by mobiles phones, as a means to build and maintain trust. These communicative practices were hardly static, being highly dependent on the situation, and importantly, the social position of the party encountered. This case study is similar to that of barefoot doctors at the margins of the healthcare system in China (Chib, Si, Hway, & Phuong, 2013), who utilized mobile phones to negotiate professional relationships depending on the social capital therein. While such a Western theory could well describe the phenomenon encountered, the Chinese cultural concept of *guanxi* provides far greater explanatory power and deeper insights. We find that *guanxi* relations describe the power hierarchies of rural barefoot doctors vis-à-vis their urban counterparts, who as the insider network, have greater medical knowledge, access to health resources, and comprise the formal healthcare information system (HIS). Rural doctors then utilize mobile phones in a parallel *guanxi* system using their existing social networks. The Chinese concept of social relations thus provides us insights into barriers faced in implementation of HIS. Further, the concept can be incorporated into program design for interventionary programs that minimize top-down centralized control in favor of more participatory designs that give voice to the margins. The implications from the cautionary tale of *guanxi* mimics the recommendations of Watkins and Baulch (Chap. 4) to pay attention to the sociocultural contexts of mHealth implementations.

In Chap. 7, Chen examines mHealth apps, having gained popularity in China with the proliferation of smartphones, and finds that levels of app integration into lifestyles and perceptions of the role of apps vary between users. Users have differing comfort levels and knowledge of how the apps work, leading to different usage patterns. In the intrapersonal sphere, while some users appreciated how apps gave them greater control over their health, others were worried about being over-dependent on apps. In the social sphere, mHealth apps gave users a sense of belonging to a larger community with similar health pursuits, but also caused some to feel lonely as apps facilitated exercise conducted in isolation. Chen proposes that app developers take into consideration how to empower users to feel in control of their health regime, and integrate them into a larger health community through social features in the app. Krömer (2016) argues that few mHealth projects have applied the theoretical concept of empowerment, with existing theories relating to either personal or psychological motivations. There is an opportunity to develop culturally relevant theorizing to integrate empowerment with social influences from a Chinese (Asian) perspective.

In conclusion, one might very well ask whether the 'hard scholarly evidence', the lack of which our editors lament, has been indeed discovered. We would do well to pause before making judgments about evidence of impact, given the range of illustrations available, and the respective lenses that varied stakeholders will use to examine the evidence base. The contribution of this volume is to argue for the application of a sociocultural structural lens to issues of power within complex and variegated societies which applies beyond that of the mHealth domain. This set of empirical and conceptual contributions provides such a lens, allowing us to shift the needle just that bit forward. This collection is exemplary in bringing a range of (new) voices in mHealth in Asia to the fore. The discipline can only gain from the increased research capacities and the growing body of sophisticated analysis and evidence.

References

Agarwal, S., Perry, H. B., Long, L. A., & Labrique, A. B. (2015). Evidence on feasibility and effective use of mHealth strategies by frontline health workers in developing countries: systematic review. *Tropical Medicine and International Health, 20*(8), 1003–1014.

Blynn, E., & Aubuchon, J. (2009). *Piloting mHealth: A research scan.* Cambridge, MA: Knowledge Exchange. Retrieved from https://wiki.brown.edu/confluence/download/attachments/9994241/mHealth+Final.pdf.

Chib, A. (2013). The promise and perils of mHealth in developing countries. *Mobile Media and Communication, 1*(1), 69–75.

Chib, A., & Chen, V. H. H. (2011). Midwives with mobiles: A dialectical perspective on gender arising from technology introduction in rural Indonesia. *New Media and Society, 12*(3), 486–501.

Chib, A., Lwin, M. O., Ang, J., Lin, H., & Santoso, F. (2008). Midwives and mobiles: Using ICTs to improve healthcare in Aceh Besar Indonesia. *Asian Journal of Communication, 18*(4), 348–364.

Chib, A., Si, C. W., Hway, N. S., & Phuong, T. K. (2013a). Enabling informal digital "guanxi" for rural doctors in Shaanxi China. *Chinese Journal of Communication, 6*(1), 1–19.

Chib, A., Wilkin, H., & Hoefman, B. (2013b). Vulnerabilities in mHealth implementation: Ugandan HIV/AIDS SMS campaign. *Global Health Promotion, 20*(Supp. 1), 26–32.

Chib, A., Wilkin, H., Leow, X. L., Hoefman, B., & van Bejima, H. (2012). Evaluating the effectiveness of a text message HIV/AIDS campaign in North West Uganda. *Journal of Health Communication, 17*(sup1), 146–157.

Chib, A., van Velthoven, M., & Car, J. (2014). mHealth adoption in low-resource environments: A review of the use of mobile healthcare in developing countries. *Journal of Health Communication, 20*(1), 4–34.

Cole-Lewis, H., & Kershaw, T. (2010). Text messaging as a tool for behavior change in disease prevention and management. *Epidemiology Review, 32*(1), 56–69.

Crenshaw, K. (1989). Demarginalizing the intersection of race and sex: A black feminist critique of antidiscrimination doctrine, feminist theory and antiracist politics. *University of Chicago Legal Forum, 1989*(1), Article 8.

Deglise, C., Suggs, L. S., & Odermatt, P. (2012). Short message service (SMS) applications for disease prevention in developing countries. *Journal of Medical Internet Research, 14*(1), e3.

Fjeldsoe, B. S., Marshall, A. L., & Miller, Y. D. (2009). Behavior change interventions delivered by mobile telephone short-message service. *American Journal of Preventive Medicine, 36*(2), 165–173.

Fry, J. P., & Neff, R. A. (2009). Periodic prompts and reminders in health promotion and health intervention behaviour interventions: Systematic review. *Journal of Medical Internet Research, 11*(2), e16.

Gurman, T. A., Rubin, S. E., & Roess, A. A. (2012). Effectiveness of mHealth behavior change communication interventions in developing countries: A systematic review of the literature. *Journal of Health Communication, 17*(Suppl. 1), 82–104.

Gurol-Urganci, I., de Jongh, T., Vodopivec-Jamsek, V., Car, J., & Atun, R. (2012). Mobile phone messaging for communicating results of medical investigations. *Cochrane Database of Systematic Reviews, 6,* CD007456.

Guy, R., Hocking, J., Wand, H., Stott, S., Ali, H., & Kaldor, J. (2012). How effective are short message service reminders at increasing clinic attendance? A meta-analysis and systematic review. *Health Services Research, 47,* 614–632.

Higgs, E. S., Goldberg, A. B., Labrique, A. B., Cook, S. H., Schmid, C., Cole, C. F., et al. (2014). Understanding the role of mHealth and other media interventions for behavior change to enhance child survival and development in low-and middle-income countries: An evidence review. *Journal of Health Communication, 19*(sup1), 164–189.

Klasnja, P., & Pratt, W. (2012). Healthcare in the pocket: Mapping the space of mobile phone health interventions. *Journal of Biomedical Informatics, 45,* 184–198.

Krishna, S., Boren, S. A., & Balas, E. A. (2009). Healthcare via cell phones: A systematic review. *Telemedicine Journal and E-Health, 15*(3), 231–240.

Krömer, N. (2016, June). *Patient empowerment through diabetes app usage and perceived app utility for diabetes management in Singapore.* Presentation at the all-powerful mobile 13th International Communication Association Mobile Pre-Conference, Fukuoka, Japan.

Mechael, P., Batavia, N., Kaonga, N., Searle, S., Kwan, A., Goldberger, A., & Ossman, J. (2010). Barriers and gaps affecting m-Health in low and middle income countries. Policy White Paper. New York, NY: Center for Global Health and Economic Development, Earth Institute, Columbia University.

Nguyen, H., Chib, A., & Mahalingam, R. (2017). Mobile phones and gender empowerment: Negotiating the essentialist-aspirational dialectic. *Information Technologies and International Development [Special Section], 13,* 170–184.

Patrick, K., Griswold, W. G., Raab, F., & Intille, S. S. (2008). Health and the mobile phone. *American Journal of Preventive Medicine, 35,* 177–181.

Tomlinson, M., Rotheram-Borus, M. J., Swartz, L., & Tsai, A. C. (2013). Scaling up mHealth: Where is the evidence? *PLoS medicine, 10*(2), e1001382.

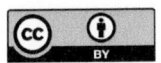